Complications in Hand Surgery

Guest Editor

JEFFREY A. GREENBERG, MD, MS

HAND CLINICS

www.hand.theclinics.com

May 2010 • Volume 26 • Number 2

SAUNDERS an imprint of ELSEVIER, Inc.

W.B. SAUNDERS COMPANY
A Division of Elsevier Inc.

1600 John F. Kennedy Blvd. • Suite 1800 • Philadelphia, Pennsylvania 19103

http://www.theclinics.com

HAND CLINICS Volume 26, Number 2
May 2010 ISSN 0749-0712, ISBN-13: 978-1-4377-1825-6

Editor: Debora Dellapena

Hand Clinics (ISSN 0749-0712) is published quarterly by Elsevier Inc., 360 Park Avenue South, New York, NY 10010-1710. Months of publication are February, May, August, and November. Business and Editorial Offices: 1600 John F. Kennedy Blvd., Ste. 1800, Philadelphia, PA 19103-2899. Customer Service Office: 3251 Riverport Lane, Maryland Heights, MO 63043. Periodicals postage paid at New York, NY and at additional mailing offices. Subscription price is $316.00 per year (domestic individuals), $491.00 per year (domestic institutions), $161.00 per year (domestic students/residents), $360.00 per year (Canadian individuals), $561.00 per year (Canadian institutions), $429.00 per year (international individuals), $561.00 per year (international institutions), and $212.00 per year (international and Canadian students/residents). Foreign air speed delivery is included in all *Clinics* subscription prices. All prices are subject to change without notice. **POSTMASTER:** Send address changes to *Hand Clinics*, Elsevier Health Sciences Division, Subscription Customer Service, 3251 Riverport Lane, Maryland Heights, MO 63043. Customer Service (orders, claims, online, change of address): Elsevier Health Sciences Division, Subscription Customer Service, 3251 Riverport Lane, Maryland Heights, MO 63043. Tel: 1-800-654-2452 (U.S. and Canada); 314-447-8871 (outside U.S. and Canada). Fax: 314-447-8029. E-mail: journalscustomerservice-usa@elsevier.com (for print support); journalsonlinesupport-usa@elsevier.com (for online support).

Reprints. For copies of 100 or more of articles in this publication, please contact the Commercial Reprints Department, Elsevier Inc., 360 Park Avenue South, New York, New York 10010-1710. Tel.: 212-633-3812; Fax: 212-462-1935; E-mail: reprints@elsevier.com.

Hand Clinics is covered in *MEDLINE/PubMed (Index Medicus), Current Contents/Clinical Medicine, EMBASE/Excerpta Medica,* and *ISI/BIOMED.*

Printed and bound by CPI Group (UK) Ltd, Croydon, CR0 4YY

Transferred to Digital Print 2011

Contributors

GUEST EDITOR

JEFFREY A. GREENBERG, MD, MS
Indiana Hand to Shoulder Center; Clinical
Assistant Professor, Department of Orthopedic
Surgery, Indiana University, Indianapolis,
Indiana

AUTHORS

BRIAN D. ADAMS, MD
Professor, Department of Orthopaedic
Surgery, University of Iowa Hospitals and
Clinics, Iowa City, Iowa

CHRISTOPHER H. ALLAN, MD
Associate Professor, Department of
Orthopaedics and Sports University of
Washington, Seattle, Washington

AJAY K. BALARAM, MD
Senior Resident, Department of Orthopaedic
Surgery and Rehabilitation, Stritch School of
Medicine, Loyola University Chicago,
Maywood, Illinois

MARK BARATZ, MD
Director, Division of Hand and Upper
Extremity Surgery; Vice Chairman,
Department of Orthopaedic Surgery,
Allegheny General Hospital; Professor,
Department of Orthopaedic Surgery,
Drexel University College of Medicine,
Philadelphia; Division Director, Allegheny
General Hospital of Upper Extremity
Surgery; Director, Allegheny General
Hospital Orthopedic Residency and
Fellowship Programs, Pittsburgh, Pennsylvania

MICHAEL S. BEDNAR, MD
Chief, Division of Hand Surgery; Professor,
Department of Orthopaedic Surgery and
Rehabilitation, Stritch School of Medicine,
Loyola University Chicago, Maywood, Illinois

JAMES CHANG, MD
Chief, Division of Plastic and Reconstructive
Surgery; Professor of Surgery (Plastic Surgery)
and Orthopedic Surgery, Hand and
Microsurgery, Stanford University Medical
Center, Palo Alto, California

MARK S. COHEN, MD
Professor; Director, Orthopaedic Education;
Director, Hand and Elbow Section,
Department of Orthopaedic Surgery, Rush
University; Midwest Orthopaedics at Rush,
Chicago, Illinois

DAMIEN I. DAVIS, MD
Fellow, Division of Hand and Upper Extremity
Surgery, Allegheny General Hospital,
Pittsburgh, Pennsylvania

CPT MATTHEW L. DRAKE, MD
Fellow, The Curtis National Hand Center,
Union Memorial Hospital, Baltimore,
Maryland; Walter Reed Army Medical Center,
Washington, DC

R. GLENN GASTON, MD
Chief of Hand Surgery, Carolinas Medical
Centre; OrthoCarolina, Charlotte, North
Carolina

EMILY GRAUEL, MS
Division of Plastic and Reconstructive Surgery,
Stanford University Medical Center, Palo Alto,
California

DOUGLAS P. HANEL, MD
Professor, Department of Orthopaedics and Sports Medicine, University of Washington, Seattle, Washington

F. THOMAS D. KAPLAN, MD
Clinical Assistant Professor of Orthopaedic Surgery, Indiana Hand to Shoulder Center, Indianapolis, Indiana

LEO I. KATOLIK, MD
Assistant Professor, Department of Orthopaedic Surgery, Thomas Jefferson University School of Medicine, Philadelphia, Pennsylvania

WILLIAM B. KLEINMAN, MD
Senior Attending Surgeon, The Indiana Hand to Shoulder Center; Clinical Professor of Orthopaedic Surgery, Indiana University School of Medicine, Indianapolis, Indiana

L. ANDREW KOMAN, MD
Professor and Chair, Department of Orthopaedic Surgery, Wake Forest University School of Medicine, Winston-Salem, North Carolina

MARSHALL A. KUREMSKY, MD
Department of Orthopedics, Carolinas Medical Center, Charlotte, North Carolina

W.P. ANDREW LEE, MD
Professor and Chief, Division of Plastic and Reconstructive Surgery, University of Pittsburgh Medical Center, University of Pittsburgh School of Medicine, Pittsburgh, Pennsylvania

ZHONGYU LI, MD, PhD
Assistant Professor, Department of Orthopaedic Surgery, Wake Forest University School of Medicine, Winston-Salem, North Carolina

ARASH MOMENI, MD
Division of Plastic and Reconstructive Surgery, Stanford University Medical Center, Palo Alto, California

SCOTT DAVID RUHLMAN, MD
Resident, Department of Orthopaedics and Sports Medicine, University of Washington, Seattle, Washington

KEITH A. SEGALMAN, MD
Attending, The Curtis National Hand Center, Union Memorial Hospital; Assistant Professor of Orthopaedic Surgery, The Johns Hopkins School of Medicine, Baltimore, Maryland

JAIMIE T. SHORES, MD
Assistant Professor, Division of Plastic and Reconstructive Surgery, University of Pittsburgh Medical Center, University of Pittsburgh School of Medicine, Pittsburgh, Pennsylvania

BETH P. SMITH, PhD
Associate Professor, Department of Orthopaedic Surgery, Wake Forest University School of Medicine, Winston-Salem, North Carolina

THOMAS L. SMITH, PhD
Professor, Department of Orthopaedic Surgery, Wake Forest University School of Medicine, Winston-Salem, North Carolina

PETER J. STERN, MD
Hill Professor and Chairman, Department of Orthopaedic Surgery, College of Medicine, University of Cincinnati, Cincinnati, Ohio

CHRISTOPHER TUOHY, MD
Assistant Professor, Department of Orthopaedic Surgery, Wake Forest University School of Medicine, Winston-Salem, North Carolina

ROBERT W. WYSOCKI, MD
Assistant Professor, Department of Orthopaedic Surgery, Rush University; Midwest Orthopaedics at Rush, Chicago, Illinois

Contents

> Fractures of the metacarpals and phalanges represent 40% of all upper extremity fractures. Complications associated with these fractures are also prevalent, and can arise with both conservative and surgical treatment of hand fractures, making treatment of complications an essential part of caring for these injuries. In this article the treatment of complications associated with open fractures and infection are reviewed, in addition to current treatment options for malunion and stiffness.

> Management of flexor tendon injuries is one of the most demanding tasks in hand surgery. Despite substantial improvements in surgical technique and postoperative rehabilitation protocols, functional outcomes may still be somewhat unreliable. In the present article, the authors present complications encountered after flexor tendon repair and provide their preferred methods of prevention and treatment.

> The stiff finger is a frequently encountered entity in hand surgical practice. It stems from a myriad of causes, may have multiple components, and requires a variety of solutions. A true understanding of the ideal treatments for the stiff finger requires a basic understanding of the local milieu that arises from injury and the anatomic features that are at risk for pathologic changes. Hand surgeons must be able to help patients understand the various factors at play and the time course of wound healing and injury-induced inflammation, because an educated and motivated patient is the best ally in the battle against the stiff finger.

> Arthritis in the small joints of the hand can be treated with arthrodesis or arthroplasty. Arthrodesis has known risks of infection, pain, and nonunion. Distal interphalangeal (DIP) arthroplasty has been successful in preserving motion and alleviating pain for distal DIP, proximal interphalangeal, and metacarpophalangeal joints. Unfortunately, complications arise that limit the success of surgery. Silicone implants have been reliable for many years but still present with the risks of infection, implant breakage, stiffness, and pain. Newer implant designs may limit some of these

the two most recent decades, little emphasis has been placed on the great morbidity and compromise to upper limb function associated with distal radio-ulna joint (DRUJ) pathology occurring with fractures of the distal radius. This article emphasizes that attention to restoration of anatomy of the DRUJ should be considered at least as important as that given to the radio-carpal relationship. This article also points out how stiffness of forearm rotation can result from a well-treated distal radius fracture and how this complication can be treated to restore healthy upper limb function.

Postoperative infections continue to be a challenging problem. The incidence of bacterial antibiotic resistance such as methicillin-resistant *Staphylococcus aureus* is rising. There are numerous intrinsic patient factors that should be optimized before surgery to minimize the risk of surgical site infections. When postoperative infections develop, treatment must be individualized. This article outlines the principles that can help guide treatment.

Complex regional pain syndrome (CRPS) after an emergent or elective upper extremity surgery may complicate recovery, delay return to work, diminish health-related quality of life, and increase the likelihood of poor outcomes and/or litigation. CRPS after hand surgery is not uncommon and may complicate postoperative care. Early diagnosis and treatment of CRPS is critical for optimal patient outcomes. This article discusses the diagnosis, physiology, and management of postsurgical CRPS that occurs after hand surgery.

Although many advances have been made in microsurgery, it is not without complications. As microsurgeons continue to make advances in technology, technique, and applications that expand the utility of this field to more and more patients, they must be prepared to deal with the complications related to donor and recipient sites and the medical comorbidity that accompanies these large endeavors in the pre-, post-, and intraoperative periods.

Hand Clinics

THE CLINICS ARE NOW AVAILABLE ONLINE!

Access your subscription at:
www.theclinics.com

Preface

Complications in Hand Surgery

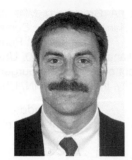

Jeffrey A. Greenberg, MD, MS
Guest Editor

Alone in my woodshop, threateningly close to razor-sharp carbide and steel moving faster than 100 miles per hour, I am constantly aware of a potential "complication." An error in technique, rushing to get done, or skipping a step in my mental safety checklist could ruin a valuable piece of wood, or, more seriously, a piece of my extremity, which could possibly threaten my career. The wood is easily replaced. I can start all over. Hopefully, by following strict safety protocols, bodily damage will not occur.

Complications in the woodshop are inevitable. They may be due to errors in planning, execution, or technique. The same holds true for complications in hand surgery. Despite the best planning and intentions, complications occur. In his book entitled, *Complications*, Atul Gawande, speaking from a general surgeon's perspective, he states, "we look for medicine to be an orderly field of knowledge and procedure but it is not. It is an enterprise of constantly changing knowledge, uncertain information, fallible individuals, and at the same time lives on the line. There is science in what we do, yes, but also habit, intuition, and sometimes plain old guessing. The gap between what we know and we aim for persists. This gap complicates everything we do."

Complications are a certainty in any surgical field and the specialty of hand surgery is no exception. In putting together this issue of *Hand Clinics*, I tried to assemble a series of topics whose complications have touched the lives of many hand surgeons. These are not esoteric topics but ones that all practicing hand surgeons can expect to encounter in the course of their careers.

It is unfortunate that complications are so misunderstood. To the lay public, the media, and certainly legal professionals, complications always have a root cause. To these groups, the root cause is a bad or negligent physician. Public and nonmedical professionals do not understand the complex environment that physicians work in and the innumerable factors considered when making medical and surgical decisions. Some of these factors are uncontrollable and random, and their effects on outcomes and results are unpredictable. Complications are a part of practices and as such should be used educationally. Those who are fortunate enough to have practices that include morbidity and mortality conferences are lucky, because in an open fashion with colleagues and partners complications are discussed and experiences with them are used to refine and change technique and practice. In the current state of medicine, complications are too often shielded, shrouded in shame, and not critically analyzed. They should be embraced.

In this issue, I have assembled a group of colleagues and friends who are recognized experts in their fields. The articles are diverse and cover a wide range of common clinical topics. This group of authors has experienced complications in their own clinical practices, and it is my

Hand Clin 26 (2010) ix–x
doi:10.1016/j.hcl.2010.03.001

hand.theclinics.com

hope that readers will use the authors' experiences to minimize complications in their own practices. I personally thank each of them for their efforts put forth for this issue. In addition, I have asked my friend and colleague, Dr Peter Stern, to add commentary regarding complications. Peter has, in his career, never been bashful about publishing articles on complications, and his presentations and lectures always contain his personal clinical cases that have not gone as predicted. I have always been impressed with Peter's ability to use his personal case complications as teaching points. Reflections on these cases have been extremely instructive. I thank him for his personal contribution as well.

Finally, I need to thank my most loyal supporters— Nancy, who has been with me on this wild ride since the beginning, and Ryann and Sawyer whom I am so proud of. They are the best back-up team that anyone can ask for.

Jeffrey A. Greenberg, MD, MS
Indiana Hand to Shoulder Center
8501 Harcourt Road
Indianapolis, IN 46260, USA
Department of Orthopedic Surgery
Indiana University, Indianapolis, IN, USA

E-mail address:
JAG@hand.md

Editorial

Complications in Hand Surgery

Complications are the bane of any surgeon's existence. They are no doubt under-reported because permanent injury is rare; some surgeons view them as unusual events; surgeons are viewed as infallible; and there is a fear of malpractice litigation.

Nearly a century ago, E.A. Codman, MD, a young Harvard surgeon, recognized the importance of complications in improving patient care. He publicly challenged his entrenched, senior colleagues by posting operative complications in the lobby of the Massachusetts General Hospital (MGH). Ultimately, this led to his dismissal from the MGH medical staff. He then established his own hospital across town and had a most distinguished career. His legacy was the end-result concept in the form of the country's first sarcoma registry, which tracked survival rates after treatment for sarcomas over time.

When analyzing complications, 2 terms are applicable, *error* and *complication*. An error is an unintended act of omission or commission—that is, an event that is preventable presumably by more education and diligence. Examples of errors include

- A carpal fracture/dislocation due to misinterpretation of plain radiographs (strictly speaking, this is an error rather than a complication)
- Simulators of infection, such as gout, which can lead to an unnecessary surgical procedure
- Pathologic fractures, which, when missed, can have catastrophic consequences.

A true complication, alternatively, is usually unavoidable (eg, a postoperative infection).

In surgery, errors and complications are more likely to occur in certain settings. Fatigue can lead to sloppy decision making or poor surgical technique, especially when performing microsurgery. Rushed treatment, such as taking shortcuts to get to a busy office or important meeting, is inexcusable but I am sure happens frequently. Finally, a small percentage of surgeons suffer from substance abuse. Help, in the form of intervention, is available in every state but probably underutilized.

Errors and complications can never be fully prevented. There are several things, however, that can be done to minimize them.

- Practice: surgical skill and proficiency comes with practice. Surgeons must take advantage of the many workshops professional organizations offer.
- Continuing medical education: hand surgery is constantly changing. Professional societies, books, and journals must be regularly used to stay on top of a specialty.
- Observe strict protocols, such as signing site and time out before surgery.
- Death and complications conference: from my perspective, this is a must, regardless of practice setting. Surgeons can learn from mistakes, and, hopefully, by presenting them to colleagues, minimize their recurrence.

Goethe, in *Maxims and Reflections*, captured the essence of the best approach to errors:

The most fruitful lesson is the conquest of one's own error. Whoever refuses to admit error may be a great scholar, but he is not a great learner. Whoever is ashamed of error will struggle against recognizing and admitting it, which means that he struggles against his greatest inward gain.

Peter J. Stern, MD
Department of Orthopaedic Surgery
College of Medicine, University of Cincinnati
231 Albert Sabin Way
5508 MSB, PO Box 670212
Cincinnati, OH 45267-0212, USA

E-mail address:
pstern@handsurg.com

Hand Clin 26 (2010) xi
doi:10.1016/j.hcl.2010.03.002
0749-0712/10/$ – see front matter © 2010 Elsevier Inc. All rights reserved.

Complications After the Fractures of Metacarpal and Phalanges

Ajay K. Balaram, MD, Michael S. Bednar, MD*

KEYWORDS

- Metacarpals • Phalanges • Complications
- Fractures • Open • Treatment

Fractures of the metacarpals and phalanges are common injuries, representing 40% of all upper extremity fractures.[1] Unfortunately, complications associated with these fractures are also prevalent, making treatment of such complications an essential part of caring for these injuries. Complications can arise with both conservative and surgical treatment of hand fractures. Closed treatment of fractures with immobilization can lead to malunion and stiffness.[2] Surgical treatment of unstable fractures adds the potential for hardware-related adhesions, tendon rupture, and infection.[2–4] Further treatment pitfalls can occur with the addition of open fractures and soft tissue injury to the hand and fingers.

Green[2] and later Creighton and Steichen[5] have written on complications of metacarpal and phalangeal fractures in previous editions of *Hand Clinics*. Green reviewed treatment of malunion and nonunion, and Creighton and Steichen have reported extensively on extensor tenolysis to address stiffness associated with these fractures. The treatment of complications associated with open fractures and infection are reviewed here in addition to current treatment options for malunion and stiffness.

OPEN FRACTURES

Open fractures of the hand are associated with injuries to the surrounding soft tissue. These fractures often involve injury to neurovascular structures or tendons. The incidence of open injuries has been reported to be as high as 34% to 68% of hand fractures.[6] The extent of soft tissue damage is directly correlated with the functional outcome for the patient.[6–8] The proper treatment of these fractures is based on the central tenets of early antibiotic administration, irrigation and debridement, stabilization, and soft tissue coverage. Rates of complications for infection, stiffness, nonunion, and malunion are all increased in open fractures.[6,8]

Classification

Open fractures of long bones have routinely been classified using the Gustilo and Anderson classification system.[9] This system is based on the size of laceration associated with the fracture and progressive soft tissue compromise. Open hand fractures and their outcomes do not necessarily correlate with this system, and attempts have been made to devise a classification system that incorporates concerns unique to the hands.

Swanson and colleagues[8] retrospectively reviewed open hand fractures and classified them based on clean versus contaminated and delay to treatment. Type I fractures are clean with no delay in treatment in a systemically well patient, and type II are contaminated or have a delay in treatment greater than 24 hours. The data showed a significant increase in infection rate when comparing type I to type II fractures (1.4% vs

Department of Orthopaedic Surgery and Rehabilitation, Stritch School of Medicine, Loyola University – Chicago, Maguire Center, Suite 1700, 2160 South, 1st Avenue, Maywood, IL 60153, USA
* Corresponding author.
E-mail address: mbednar@lumc.edu

Hand Clin 26 (2010) 169–177
doi:10.1016/j.hcl.2010.01.005
0749-0712/10/$ – see front matter. Published by Elsevier Inc.

14%). Although this classification is basic, it demonstrates the importance of early treatment for improved outcomes.

McLain and colleagues[10] and later, Duncan and colleagues[7] modified the Gustilo and Anderson classification by downscaling the system to apply to fractures associated with the hands. McLain described type I fractures as clean wounds with smaller than 1-cm lacerations with no crush of skin or comminution of bone. Type II fractures were those with clean lacerations greater than 1 cm with no fracture comminution. Type III injuries had lacerations greater than 1 cm with contamination of the wound, soft tissue crush, comminuted fractures, or periosteal stripping. Duncan further subcategorized type III injuries to include lacerations greater than 2 cm or gross contamination (IIIA), periosteal stripping or elevation (IIIB), and associated neurovascular injury (IIIC). The familiarity of the orthopedic surgeon with the original Gustilo classification makes the modified classification devised by McLain and Duncan a reproducible and useful system to dictate treatment and predict outcomes.

Infection

Open fractures of the hand have shown an overall deep infection rate of 2% to 11%,[6,10] compared with an infection rate of less than 0.5% in closed fractures undergoing operative intervention. The rate of infection is directly correlated to the soft tissue involvement and contamination of the wound.[6-8,10] Gram-positive cocci, such as *Staphylococcus* and *Streptococcus*, are the most common bacteria isolated from open hand fractures. Human and animal bite wounds can produce mixed flora infections that routinely include *Eikenella* and *Pasteurella* species, respectively. Farm injuries have a high incidence of gram-negative bacteria. Antibiotic treatment of open fractures should provide broad coverage initially based on mechanism of injury. Cultures should be taken during the initial debridement and coverage should be tailored to the specified bacterium.

Timing of Treatment

An emergent operative debridement of open fractures is generally recommended to prevent infection. Timing to treatment of open hand fractures should be done urgently, but evidence has shown emergent treatment may not alter the outcomes for every open fracture class. Data to support early (within 6 hours) treatment of open hand fractures is not evident in the literature. McLain and colleagues[10] showed no increased incidence of infection in open hand fractures, regardless of grade, treated after 12 hours from injury when compared with those with no delay in treatment. This finding is contradictory to the earlier held belief that open hand fractures should be addressed in the 6 hours immediately after the injury occurs. Although each case must be evaluated separately, this potentially obviates the need for emergent operative intervention for these fractures. In certain open fractures, evidence allows for cases to be addressed during routine operative time on the morning after the injury. Regardless of time to surgery, prophylactic antibiotics and an adequate irrigation and immobilization of these injuries must occur on evaluation in the emergency department.

TREATMENT OF OPEN FRACTURES

The treatment of open fractures is based on an aggressive attempt to prevent complications that are so common in these injuries. Gonzales and colleagues[11] published an algorithm for treatment of open fractures based on the modified Gustilo classification of these injuries. The aim is to address open fractures in a systematic manner to prevent infection and other potential complications. Type I injuries are treated as an operative closed injury, with 24 hours of cefazolin or clindamycin, irrigation, debridement, and primary closure of wound. Fractures can be treated closed or with plate fixation, or percutaneously pinned. Extending the open wound for fixation should be done with caution as this extension has been shown to increase complications, essentially transforming a type I injury into a type IIIB injury.[7] Predicting whether an injury is type II or III can be difficult in the emergency room because the amount of soft tissue stripping and deep contamination may not be appreciated by inspection alone. For type II injuries, Gonzales and colleagues recommend treating these fractures operatively with irrigation and debridement, stabilizing the fractures with K-wires or external fixators, leaving the wounds open or loosely closed, and performing a second look debridement at 24 to 72 hours post injury. Intravenous antibiotics are continued for 72 hours. If during the second look the wound is clean, definitive fixation can be performed. If infection is present, these injuries are treated as a type III wound. Others would argue that a true type II injury does not have significant soft tissue stripping or contamination and should be definitively fixed during the initial debridement. For type III injuries, penicillin should be added if there is gross soil contamination. Here, there is little argument that the patient should be taken to the operating room for aggressive debridement and fracture fixation initially performed with either K-wires or external fixation. A second-look debridement should be performed within 24 to 72 hours and re-debrided as necessary thereafter. Quantitative cultures should be taken with each debridement and fixation or coverage withheld until bacterial counts drop to less than 10^5 per gram. Soft tissue coverage with a flap or graft should ideally be performed within a week to prevent secondary bacterial contamination.

Osteomyelitis

Infection of the bones of the hand is a potentially devastating complication of open hand fractures and penetrating injuries. Osteomyelitis is defined as a pyogenic infection of bone, usually caused by a direct inoculation of bacteria in the tubular bones of the hand. Although a rare complication of open fracture, osteomyelitis can have demoralizing outcomes, with more than 50% going on to amputation.[12] Diagnosis is based on clinical examination and plain radiographs, with advanced imaging being of little added benefit (**Fig. 1**).[13] Diagnosis is only confirmed after bone biopsy and positive cultures from the offending sequestrum. Once the diagnosis is made, nonoperative treatment is of little value. In the setting of fracture and osteomyelitis, the following 2-stage treatment protocol is performed.

After diagnosis, all implants are removed from the affected bone. Both soft tissue and bone cultures are taken intraoperatively. A debridement of infected soft tissue and bone is performed until bleeding viable bone is exposed. Antibiotic impregnated methyl methacrylate spacers are placed into the defect, and external or internal fixation is placed before wound closure. Fixation at this juncture is important to allow motion and prevent stiffness of uninvolved joints during this staged treatment. When cultures are positive, culture-specific antibiotics are started. Otherwise empirical treatment is based on the most likely cause of infection. Infectious disease consultation is recommended. Antibiotics are continued for 4 to 6 weeks postoperatively, and after this course is finished the patient is given a period of 4 weeks free of antibiotics to allow any residual infection to surface. If the patient remains asymptomatic and clinical laboratory markers including erythrocyte sedimentation rate and C-reactive protein have returned to normal, the patient is taken to the operating room for the second stage of the procedure. At this time, cultures are taken intraoperatively and sent for frozen sections. If no infectious material is present, the bone cement is

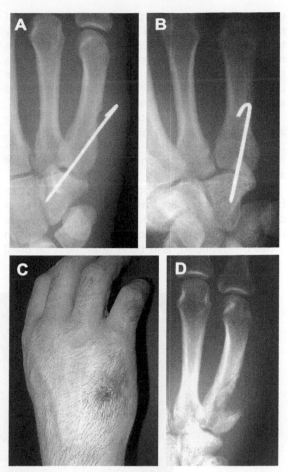

Fig. 1. Osteomyelitis after pinning. (*A, B*) Pinning of ring: small carpometacarpal dislocation. (*C*) Drainage from pin site. (*D*) Radiograph taken after pin removal. (*D*) Hypertrophic nonunion.

removed and autologous grafting with internal fixation is performed.

Nonunion

Nonunion after metacarpal and phalangeal fractures is a rare complication, frequently associated with concurrent soft tissue injury. Nonunions are often found in the setting of nerve injury, infection, and bone loss. Complex open fractures or a devascularizing approach to fixation can also lead to nonunion. Jupiter and colleagues[14] defined nonunion and delayed unions together as those fractures without clinical or radiographic evidence of healing at 4 months after the initial injury. The radiographic evidence of nonunion alone is usually insufficient, as radiographic fracture lines can be present up to 14 months after fracture.[15] Clinical evidence of pain is also unreliable, as many fractures are associated with nerve damage and stiffness that can cause pain. The combination of radiographic and clinical signs is the optimal way to diagnose nonunion. Similar to long bones, the nonunion classification of Weber and Cech can be attributed to hand fractures. These fractures can be defined as hypertrophic or atrophic, and similar treatment principles apply.

In hypertrophic nonunions, stability is often lacking and can result from inadequate immobilization, soft tissue interposition, or failed fixation. Treatment of this uncommon hand injury consists of stable fixation (**Fig. 2**).

Atrophic nonunions occur more frequently as bone loss from penetrating injuries or infection compromises bony apposition (**Fig. 3**). In these cases the fibrous interposing tissues or infection must be debrided, and bone graft must be used to bridge any bone deficiency. Stable fixation techniques can allow for early range of motion and prevention of joint stiffness. Prolonged immobilization is contraindicated in the treatment of nonunions to prevent stiffness. Tenolysis is often needed after surgical treatment of nonunion to improve functional results.[16,17]

Results of surgery for nonunion are sparse in the literature. The series of Smith and Rider[15] has shown that results with bone graft and plate fixation have been superior to Kirschner wire fixation for nonunions. In this study, even optimal treatment resulted in few well-functioning digits. Treatment of nonunion in an insensate digit or with severe soft tissue loss is rarely indicated. Even if bony union is achieved, a nonfunctional digit is a continued liability to the function of the hand.[16]

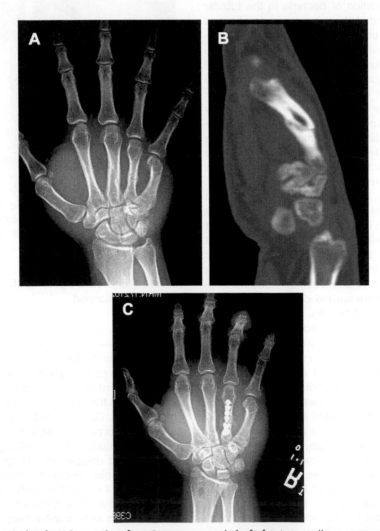

Fig. 2. (*A*) Radiograph taken 3 months after ring metacarpal shaft fracture; callous seen around fracture. (*B*) Computed tomography scan showing nonunion. (*C*) Treatment with debridement of nonunion and rigid internal fixation.

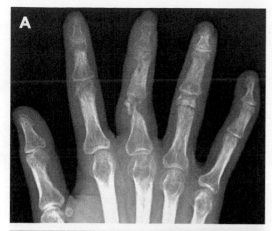

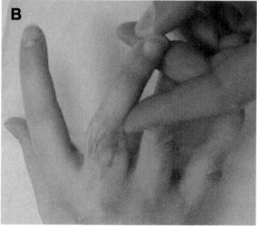

Fig. 3. (*A*) Radiograph of open fracture. (*B*) Nonunion diagnosis after open fracture.

In this setting amputation may provide the best outcome for the patient.

Malunion

Malunion after metacarpal and phalangeal fractures is the most common complication encountered after injury. Deformity can be in the form of shortening, rotation, or angular malalignment. Malunion is usually evident after closed treatment of unstable fractures, but can also arise after failed open reduction and internal fixation. In addition to negative functional effects, deformity may be cosmetically unappealing as well. Although guidelines have been developed to address surgical correction for malunion, treatment must be patient specific; indications must consider patients' vocational and avocational interests and activities, as well as expectations.

METACARPAL

Deforming forces acting on metacarpal fractures often lead to a shortening of the digit after spiral and oblique fractures. Shortening of the digit can alter the intricate balance of digital motion supplied by the extrinsic and intrinsic systems. Extensor tendon dysfunction is more likely than flexor tendon or interosseous muscle dysfunction after shortening of a metacarpal. Strauch and colleagues[18] have demonstrated a 7° extensor lag for every 2 mm of shortening found in metacarpal fractures. The ability of the metacarpophalangeal (MCP) joints to hyperextend on average 20° allows for functionality with some extensor lag. Therefore, a conclusion is drawn that 6 mm of shortening (21° extensor lag) is acceptable, as hyperextension can maintain motion to full extension. With greater than 6 mm of shortening, open reduction and internal fixation should be performed to reduce shortened oblique and spiral metacarpal fractures.

Angular Malunion

Angular malunion can exist in either the sagittal plane or coronal plane, and can cause both functional and cosmetic deficits. Metacarpal shaft fractures are generally angulated in the sagittal plane with an apex dorsal deformity. Acceptable angulation is debatable, but safe ranges allowing normal function range from 10° (index and middle fingers) to 20° (ring fingers) to 30° (small finger).[18] This range reflects the ability of the ring and small finger carpometacarpal joints to compensate for functional loss due to angulation. Often there is a mixed deformity including sagittal and coronal plane deformity; coronal plane is less tolerable and should be corrected if malunion results in angulation of the digit on examination.

Rotational Deformity

Although angular deformity can be compensated by adjacent joint motion, rotational malunion transmits deformity distally to affect the entire digit. For this reason rotational deformity is unacceptable in metacarpal malunion. Evaluation is made with the patient making a fist while monitoring for overlap of the digits and deviance from scaphoid tubercle convergence is conducted. Study of noninjured hands has shown that the contralateral hand can be used to assess rotational deformity when comparing digit rotation and scaphoid convergence. In contrast, digital overlap of the contralateral hand may not be reliable, as there is a high probability of asymmetry between uninjured hands in the same subject.[19] A small amount of rotational malunion that is missed on initial radiographs can cause significant functional impairment, as 5° of malrotation can cause 1.5 cm of digital overlap.[20]

Correction of rotational malunion in the metacarpal can be performed at the site of the previous fracture or more proximal at the base of the affected metacarpal, as described originally by Weckesser.[21] The decision regarding where to perform the osteotomy is dependent on the concurrent angular deformity and the amount of rotation associated with the fracture. In fractures with a mixed deformity of rotation and angulation the osteotomy should be performed at the site of the fracture, as a proximal osteotomy will not address the angular deformity. In a purely rotational metacarpal shaft malunion, osteotomy can be performed at the proximal metaphysis to correct deformities up to 18° to 20° in the affected digit.[22] Fixation can be performed with crossed K-wires or plate-and-screw construct. Although the K-wire fixation may be less invasive, the plate construct can provide stability for early motion. Recent studies have focused on the step-cut osteotomy as described by Manktelow and Mahoney.[23] The step-cut osteotomy is performed at the base of the metacarpal and provides increased bony apposition for healing, and is fixed with simple lag screws thus decreasing the incidence of soft tissue adhesions associated with plate fixation.[24]

PHALANGES
Malunions

Malunions of the proximal phalanx are often categorized into 4 groups: volar angulation, lateral angulation, shortening, or rotation. Malunions are frequently multidirectional (**Fig. 4**). Apex volar angulation is common, as the intrinsic muscles flex the proximal fragment and the extensor tendon pulls proximally on the distal fragment (**Fig. 5**). Failed closed reductions can often lead to malunion. The anteroposterior view often gives a false sense of anatomic reduction, and a lateral radiograph of the isolated digit must be performed to adequately visualize reduction of the volar angulation. The shortening of the digit causes a relative extensor tendon lengthening and a subsequent extensor lag at the proximal interphalangeal (PIP) joint.[25] This extensor lag can develop into a pseudo-claw deformity of the finger as the PIP joint develops a fixed flexion contracture.

Treatment of volar angulated malunion of the proximal phalanx is best performed via a closing wedge osteotomy using the dorsal periosteum as a hinge.[2] The closing wedge osteotomy does not further affect extensor tendon function, as the dorsal length is unchanged when the volar malunion is corrected. Fixation can then be performed

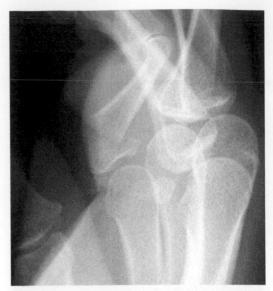

Fig. 4. Malunion of proximal phalanx proximal metaphysis fracture.

with a lateral plate to avoid dorsal tendon adhesion.

Lateral angulation of the fractured phalanx is often a result of bone loss on the affected cortex. Clinical evaluation often reveals scissoring of the digits, but can be hidden as neighboring digits are used to trap the digit during flexion into a fist. Surgical treatment is performed using an opening wedge incomplete osteotomy at the concavity of the deformity. The osteotomy should spare the far cortex at the site of the malunion, as this cortex can also be used to hinge the osteotomy open to the correct angulation.[26] Bone graft is then interposed into the defect and a lateral buttress plate is applied. New locking plates can be used laterally or dorsally. Plate fixation must provide a stable construct to start early postoperative motion. In an evaluation of osteotomies performed for bony phalangeal malunions, Büchler and colleagues[26] found a 100% union rate and excellent or good results in 96% of patients.

Intra-articular malunion presents a problem, because an extra-articular osteotomy may correct angulation but will not reduce the articular incongruity.[27] If the fracture line can be identified, an osteotomy can be performed through the articular surface and then securely fixed with a congruent articular surface.[28] Isolated arthrodesis is also an option for chronic malunions at the PIP or distal interphalangeal (DIP) but is poorly tolerated at the MCP joints. In a chronic misaligned intra-articular volar lip fracture resulting in a PIP fracture-dislocation, resection of the middle phalanx base and hemi-hamate arthroplasty has been proven

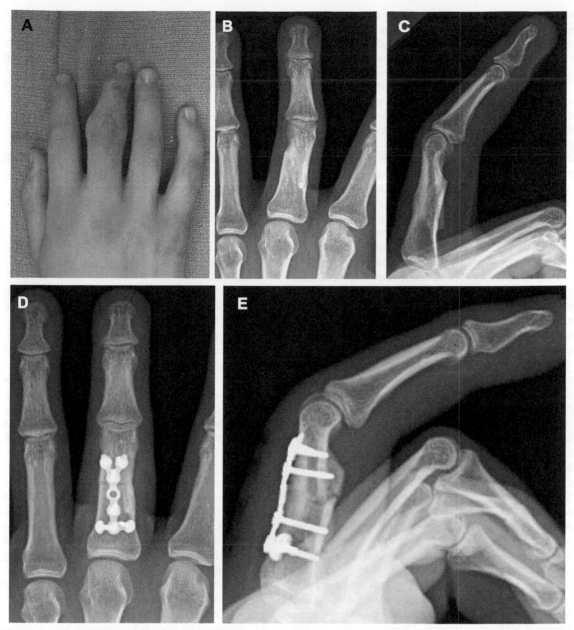

Fig. 5. (*A*) Deviation and rotation of digit. (*B*) Radiograph showing malunion. (*C–E*) Radiographs of multiplanar osteotomy with internal fixation.

to provide restoration of PIP function.[29] Other options for intra-articular malunions include osteochondral autograft and joint arthroplasty.

Stiffness

Stiffness after treatment of hand fractures is a common complication associated with tendon adhesion and immobilization. Conditions that predispose to stiffness include crush injuries, multiple finger injuries, open fractures, and immobilization longer than 4 weeks. Page and Stern[3] reported a significant decrease in loss of motion after plate fixation of phalangeal fractures as opposed to metacarpal fractures. As discussed earlier, the degree of open fracture correlates to postoperative range of motion and postoperative range of motion correlates to patient outcomes. Using total active range of motion as the outcome, Duncan and colleagues[7] reported on 140 open hand fractures. Grade I, II, and IIIA open fractures were associated with 63% good to excellent results. In contrast, grade IIIB and IIIC fractures were associated with 92% poor results. The stripping of periosteum and associated neurovascular injuries contributed to a complex injury pattern often associated with postoperative stiffness.

Principles of preventing joint stiffness are often associated with factors beyond the control of the operating room. Maximizing range of motion after fixation must be considered in the preoperative period. Although the plate-and-screw construct can provide excellent stability for early range of motion, tendon adhesions to the plate and tendon ruptures are encountered The advent of low-profile plates has increased the surgeon's options for fixation. Postoperative splinting in the safe or functional positions avoids stiffness as the MP and IP joints recover easily from flexion and extension, respectively. Close communication with hand therapists and patients concerning treatment goals are imperative to good outcomes. Edema and pain control in the early postoperative period can facilitate early motion. Active and passive range of motion and the use of dynamic splinting can optimize functional use of the hand.

Creighton and Steichen[5] have advocated extensor tenolysis and dorsal capsulotomy for decreased range of motion as a complication of phalangeal fractures. Indications include decreased active and passive flexion with maintained full extension, and a failure to improve in therapy. Soft tissue quiescence is a crucial factor to increase the effectiveness of tenolysis. Quiescence routinely requires a period of at minimum 3 months between procedures. Factors such as absence of erythema, minimal edema, and a mature scar are indicators that the soft tissues can appropriately tolerate another procedure. The technique is to elevate the central extensor tendon and lateral bands over the proximal phalanx and then release the interval between these 2 structures and the bone over the PIP joint. Elevation of the radial and ulnar portions of the terminal extensor tendon allows access to the dorsal capsule of the DIP joint. If the tenolysis alone does note achieve full active and passive range of motion, a dorsal capsulotomy can be performed. The postoperative regimen includes pain management protocols such as a transcutaneous electrical nerve stimulation unit and early range of motion, and is as important for good outcomes as the surgical procedure itself.

Surgeons who treat metacarpal and phalangeal fractures inevitably treat complications associated with these fractures. In all hand fractures the soft tissue component of the injury is directly correlated with outcomes, and should be addressed with the same attention as the fracture itself.

Outcomes have improved since the institution of stable fixation and early motion. Further investigation into improved fixation methods, soft tissue handling, and postoperative rehabilitation will provide surgeons with the chances to prevent complications in these difficult fractures.

REFERENCES

1. Chung KC, Spilson SV. The frequency and epidemiology of hand and forearm fractures in the United States. J Hand Surg 2001;26(5):908–15.
2. Green DP. Complications of phalangeal and metacarpal fractures. Hand Clin 1986;2(2):307–28.
3. Page SM, Stern PJ. Complications and range of motion following plate fixation of metacarpal and phalangeal fractures. J Hand Surg 1998;23(5): 827–32.
4. Kozin SH, Thoder JJ, Lieberman G. Operative treatment of metacarpal and phalangeal shaft fractures. J Am Acad Orthop Surg 2000;8(2):111–21.
5. Creighton JJ, Steichen JB. Complications in phalangeal and metacarpal fracture management. Results of extensor tenolysis. Hand Clin 1994;10(1):111–6.
6. Chow SP. A prospective study of 245 open digital fractures of the hand. J Hand Surg 1991;16(2): 137–40.
7. Duncan RW, Freeland AE, Jabaley ME, et al. Open hand fractures: an analysis of the recovery of active motion and complications. J Hand Surg 1993;18(3): 387–94.
8. Swanson TV, Szabo RM, Anderson MM. Open hand fractures: prognosis and classification. J Hand Surg 1991;16(1):101–7.
9. Gustillo RB, Anderson JT. Prevention of infection in the treatment of one thousand and twenty-five open fractures of long bone. J Bone Joint Surg 1976;58:453–8.
10. McLain RF, Steyers C, Stoddard M. Infections in open fractures of the hand. J Hand Surg 1991; 16(1):108–12.
11. Gonzales MH, Bach HG, Bassem TE, et al. Management of open hand fractures. J Am Soc Surg Hand 2003;3(4):208–18.
12. Reilly KE, Linz JC, Stern PJ, et al. Osteomyelitis of the tubular bones of the hand. J Hand Surg 1997; 22(4):644–9.
13. Honda H, Mcdonald JR. Current recommendations in the management of osteomyelitis of the hand and wrist. J Hand Surg 2009;34(6):1135–6.
14. Jupiter JB, Koniuch MP, Smith RJ. The management of delayed union and non-union of the metacarpals and phalanges. J Hand Surg 1985;4:457–66.
15. Smith FL, Rider DL. A study of the healing of one hundred consecutive phalangeal fractures. J Bone Joint Surg 1935;17:91–109.

16. Ring D. Malunion and non-union of the metacarpals and phalanges. Instr Course Lect 2006;55:121–8 AAOS.

17. Strauch RJ, Rosenwasser MP, Lunt JG. Metacarpal shaft fractures: the effect of shortening on the extensor tendon mechanism. J Hand Surg 1998; 23:519–23.

18. Stern PJ, Kaufman RA. Fractures of the metacarpals and phalanges. In: Green DP, Hotchkiss RN, Pederson WC, et al, editors. Green's operative hand surgery. 4th edition. Philadelphia: Elsevier Churchill Livingston; 1999. p. 277–342.

19. Tan V, Kinchelow T, Beredjiklian PK. Variation in digital rotation and alignment in normal subjects. J Hand Surg 2008;33(6):873–8.

20. Jupiter JB, Axelrod TS, Belsky MR. Fractures and dislocations of the hand. In: Browner BB, editor. Skeletal trauma. 3rd edition. Philadelphia: W.B. Saunders; 2003. p. 1153.

21. Weckesser EC. Rotational osteotomy of the metacarpal for overlapping fingers. J Bone Joint Surg 1965;47:751–6.

22. Gross MS, Gelberman RH. Metacarpal rotational osteotomy. J Hand Surg 1985;10:105–8.

23. Manktelow RT, Mahoney JL. Step osteotomy: a precise rotation osteotomy to correct scissoring deformities of the fingers. Plast Reconstr Surg 1981;68:571–6.

24. Jawa A, Zucchini M, Lauri G, et al. Modified step-cut osteotomy for metacarpal and phalangeal rotational deformity. J Hand Surg Am 2009;34:335–40.

25. Vahey, Wegner DA, Hastings H 3rd. Effect of proximal phalangeal fracture deformity on extensor tendon function. J Hand Surg 1998;23(4):673–81.

26. Büchler U, Gupta A, Ruf S. Corrective osteotomy for post-traumatic malunion of the phalanges in the hand. J Hand Surg 1996;21(1):33–42.

27. Gollamudi S, Jones WA. Corrective osteotomy of malunited fractures of phalanges and metacarpals. J Hand Surg 2000;25(5):439–41.

28. Light TL, Bednar MS. Management of intra-articular fractures of the metacarpophalangeal joint. Hand Clin 1994;10(2):303–14.

29. Calfee RP, Kiefhaber TR, Sommerkamp G, et al. Hemi-hamate arthroplasty provides functional reconstruction of acute and chronic proximal interphalangeal fracture-dislocations. J Hand Surg 2009;34:1232–41.

Complications After Flexor Tendon Injuries

Arash Momeni, MD, Emily Grauel, MS, James Chang, MD*

KEYWORDS

- Flexor tendon injury • Hand surgery • Complications

Management of flexor tendon injuries is one of the most demanding tasks in hand surgery. Despite substantial improvements in surgical technique and postoperative rehabilitation protocols, functional outcomes may still be somewhat unreliable. The treatment of flexor tendon injuries has been a controversial topic, which has produced more articles in the peer-reviewed hand surgery literature than any other single topic.[1] In particular, treatment of zone 2 injuries has been an area of great controversy since Bunnell's proposal that "it is better to remove the tendons entirely from the finger and graft in new tendons throughout its length."[2]

The challenge in the treatment of flexor tendon injuries originates from the fact that reestablishment of not only tendon continuity but also the gliding mechanism of the tendon and its surrounding structures is required for a satisfying functional outcome.[3] Pre-, intra-, and postoperative factors affect functional outcome, of which the last 2 can be influenced by the surgeon. Preoperative factors include the type of trauma (eg, cut, crush), degree of wound contamination, and associated injuries. Intraoperatively, the surgeon may influence outcome by meticulous atraumatic tissue handling along with providing a strong repair that allows for an early postoperative motion protocol.

Principles of surgical treatment of flexor tendon injuries include early primary repair (if possible) with a strong core stitch (4–6 strand) combined with an epitendinous suture. The latter, although initially thought to merely contour the repair site has been demonstrated to contribute considerably to the strength of the repair.[4] Postoperatively, an early motion protocol should be used in compliant patients to promote intrinsic healing and to minimize extrinsic scarring and adhesion formation.[5] A multitude of different protocols has been introduced[6–10]; however, the best mobilization strategy has yet to be defined.[11]

It is well known that the functional outcome of zone 2 flexor tendon injuries is poorer and is associated with a complication rate greater than that of injuries in other zones.[12] The authors' preferred method for repair of flexor tendon injuries in zone 2 is aggressive exploration and early repair on initial presentation via Bruner zigzag incisions. In the setting of injuries to both flexor tendons, every effort should be made to repair both tendons individually. Occasionally, repair of only the flexor digitorum profundus (FDP) tendon is proposed in the literature. The authors think, however, that if the flexor digitorum superficialis (FDS) tendon is left unrepaired, the free ends might contribute to excessive scar formation, with resultant functional compromise of the digit. Furthermore, repair of both tendons will still allow proximal interphalangeal (PIP) joint flexion should the repaired FDP tendon rupture during postoperative rehabilitation. Repair of both tendons also provides additional safety in the unfortunate event of rupture of 1 of the repaired tendons. During the repair, care should be taken to preserve the A2 and A4 pulleys to prevent postoperative bowstringing with resultant loss of function.

Although excellent to good outcome has been reported in more than 75% of adult and pediatric patients,[13–16] poor functional outcome continues to frustrate hand surgeons, therapists, and patients in a significant number of cases. In the present article, the authors present complications encountered after flexor tendon repair and provide

Division of Plastic and Reconstructive Surgery, Stanford University Medical Center, 770 Welch Road, Suite 400, Palo Alto, CA 94304, USA
* Corresponding author.
E-mail address: changhand@aol.com

Hand Clin 26 (2009) 179–189
doi:10.1016/j.hcl.2009.11.004
0749-0712/09/$ – see front matter. Published by Elsevier Inc.

their preferred methods of prevention and treatment.

TENDON ADHESIONS

The most common complication after surgical repair of tendon injuries is adhesion formation.[17,18] This is of particular concern in the setting of zone 2 injuries because of the unique anatomy of the flexor tendon sheath in this region. As the FDS and FDP tendons are encased in a narrow fibro-osseous tunnel, even slight bulkiness of the flexor tendon or minimal adhesion formation may result in a significant increase in friction. Thus, minimal anatomic changes within the fibro-osseous tunnel may result in marked limitation of tendon excursion and compromised function.[3] Factors that have been demonstrated to affect the formation of excursion-restricting adhesions postoperatively are trauma to the tendon and sheath from initial injury and surgical repair, tendon ischemia, immobilization, and gapping at the tendon repair site.[19]

Several strategies have been proposed to reduce adhesion formation and hence improve functional outcome. The 2 most important aspects of treatment seem to be (1) atraumatic tissue handling and (2) early postrepair motion protocols. Atraumatic tissue handling is crucial, as adhesion formation has been found to be proportional to the degree of tissue crushing and manipulation of the tendon and sheath during repair.[10,20] This explains the frequent occurrence of stiffness after crush injuries.[21] Early motion protocols postrepair have been demonstrated not only to decrease adhesion formation through improved tendon excursion and promotion of intrinsic healing but also to improve recovery of tensile strength.[22–25] Although an early motion rehabilitation program seems to be the only measure that is clinically justified in the postoperative care of patients with flexor tendon injuries, the best method of mobilization remains to be identified.[11,26]

After adequate surgical management and proper postoperative rehabilitation, several patients still experience limited range of motion (ROM) that may require further surgical intervention. Flexor tenolysis is indicated when the passive ROM is significantly greater than the active ROM.[27] Because tenolysis is the most challenging flexor tendon operation,[28] strict criteria must be met before the patient is taken to the operating room. Patient compliance, minimal joint contractures, and near-normal passive ROM must be present.[29] Furthermore, associated fractures must be well healed and the soft tissues must be soft and supple.[30]

Overall, flexor tenolysis has been reported to improve function in a significant number of patients. In a study including 78 fingers, Foucher and colleagues[31] reported an improvement in active movement from 135° to 203° in 84% of the fingers after tenolysis. Hahn and colleagues[32] reported an improvement in the total active movement from 79° to 189° in 84% of fingers treated. Eggli and colleagues[33] reviewed their series involving 23 patients and reported significant functional improvement in 88% of the digits after tenolysis.

Authors' Preferred Method

Before planning tenolysis surgery, the authors wait for a period of 3 to 6 months after tendon repair or grafting. The effects of physical therapy have typically reached a plateau after this time period. Old operative records are reviewed to see if any concomitant neurovascular injuries were repaired during the initial operation. Previous incisions are marked to prevent devascularization of skin flaps that may need to be elevated.

The procedure is ideally performed under local anesthesia with intravenous sedation, as this allows for active involvement of the patient during the procedure.[34] Despite patient participation, a proximal incision in the distal forearm may occasionally be indicated to allow traction on the tendon proximally to test for excursion. The authors prefer Bruner zigzag incisions for wide exposure,[35] which allow the best surgical exposure of the flexor tendon anatomy and pulley system.[28] Alternatively, midlateral incisions may be chosen, which leave the neurovascular bundles dorsally and are believed to reduce skin scarring directly over the flexor tendon.[28]

As anatomy may be distorted, dissection should begin in an unaffected area and proceed to the affected area.[31] Hence, normal flexor tendon should be visualized proximally and distally from the repair site. Identification and preservation of the neurovascular bundles and the borders of the flexor tendons are paramount. Also, preservation of as much of the tendon sheaths and pulley system as possible is critical for success. Blunt dissectors are used and introduced into the tendon sheath. Careful dissection is crucial to prevent injury to the overlying pulleys. An Allis clamp is then placed around the normal tendon proximally and twirled to allow axial tension on the tendon without the risk of causing pulley rupture (**Fig. 1A–C**). Fine blunt scissors may be used within the tunnel to release any remaining adhesions. Occasionally, the repaired FDS may

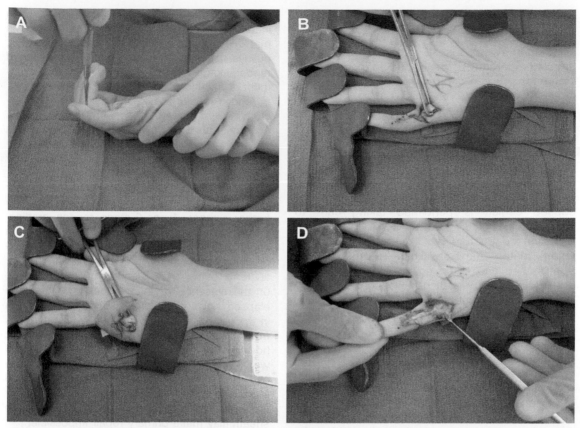

Fig. 1. Authors' preferred method for flexor tenolysis. (*A*) Preoperative image demonstrating limited passive extension secondary to adhesions. (*B*) An Allis clamp is placed around the tendon. Note that the tendon is not crushed. (*C*) As the Allis clamp is twirled, axial tension is placed on the tendon without the risk of causing pulley rupture. (*D*) Full passive extension after flexor tendon tenolysis.

need to be excised to allow free gliding of the more critical FDP tendon.

Full passive ROM should be achieved intraoperatively, as motion will only decrease during the postoperative period as a result of tissue edema and scar formation (**Fig. 1**D). Once full passive ROM is achieved, the wounds should be closed. Immediate active and passive ROM exercises should be resumed postoperatively to maintain the gains achieved after tenolysis.

The complexity of tenolysis is reflected by the set of possible complications, such as pain, prolonged edema, and inadvertent injury to the neurovascular bundles. Furthermore, the operation may fail to improve ROM and, in fact, may result in worsening of finger function. Also, tendon rupture may occur after tenolysis. This would require staged flexor tendon reconstruction as a salvage procedure.

JOINT CONTRACTURE

Despite optimal surgical management, functional outcome is compromised by the occurrence of joint contractures in the PIP and distal interphalangeal (DIP) joints in 17% of patients.[17] However, varying degrees of joint stiffness are almost invariably present in patients after flexor tendon repair and protective motion exercise.[36] Multiple causes of joint contractures have been described, including tendon bowstringing as a result of pulley failure, injuries to the volar plate, flexor tendon adhesions, and skin contracture. The most common cause of development of joint contractures is postoperative protective finger splinting. Surgical repair itself is rarely primarily responsible for the occurrence of joint contractures. Various adjustments in the design of the protective splint have thus been proposed, including, but not limited to, placing a foam block inside the dorsal splint at the level of the proximal phalanx, which in addition to increasing metacarpophalangeal (MCP) joint flexion with subsequent relaxation of the intrinsic mechanism will help resolve PIP contracture.[37] Attention to detail when molding a splint is therefore critical in preventing significant joint contracture.

Authors' Preferred Method

Surgical release of PIP joint contractures is a straightforward task if one appreciates the detailed anatomy of the finger. In general, the cause for a flexion contracture lies volarly. Exploration and dissection should be performed in a layer-by-layer fashion until full extension of the digit is achieved. Exploration should first begin with release of any skin contracture. In the setting of skin/soft tissue deficit, placement of skin grafts or flap reconstruction may be indicated. Next, the tendon sheath should be assessed and released as necessary (**Fig. 2**A–C). Full tenolysis, as discussed earlier, is performed taking care to preserve the pulley system (**Fig. 2**D). Should a flexion contracture remain after this step the volar plate and checkrein ligaments are approached and taken down. The next step in addressing any persisting flexion contracture is releasing the collateral ligaments on both sides of the PIP joint. This typically results in full extension of the PIP joint (**Fig. 2**E, F) unless a bony block is present, which is usually diagnosed preoperatively on plain radiographs. A limitation to flexion contracture release may be excessive stretch on the neurovascular bundles in long-standing cases of flexion contracture.

The same principles outlined earlier apply to extension contractures. Again, approaching the digit from the superficial layer to deeper layers (skin, extensor tendon complex, dorsal capsule, and collateral ligaments) allows for a straightforward dissection. Preservation of the central slip of the extensor tendon as it inserts into the base of the middle phalanx is critical, as inadvertent transection or release from its insertion complicates the reconstruction and typically results in functional compromise because immediate ROM exercises are precluded in this setting. In the case of extension contracture, early surgical repair is warranted, as excessive passive physiotherapy may lead to stretching of the extensor tendon complex, a problem that is difficult to correct once it has occurred.

RUPTURE

Rupture of a tendon repair has been reported to occur in 4% to 30% of patients.[23,38–41] The most common cause for rupture is an unplanned high load that exceeds the tolerance of the repaired tendon.[15,42,43] Other predisposing factors that lead to ruptures of primary tendon repairs include poor surgical technique, poor patient compliance, overzealous therapy, and early termination of postoperative splinting.[40] Furthermore, the curvature of tendon motion affects repair strength, with an increased likelihood of repair ruptures in tendons that glide along curvatures over the sheaths, pulleys, or joints.[44] A decrease in the incidence of tendon rupture may be achieved by the establishment of practitioner-led hand therapy clinics.[45]

Tendon repairs are weakest between postoperative days 6 and 18,[46] with most ruptures occurring around day 10. However, ruptures may be seen as late as 6 to 7 weeks postoperatively.[17] Immediate repair has been traditionally advocated as the most favorable procedure[47]; however, various surgical options exist for management of a repair rupture, including no further surgery, 1- or 2-stage tendon grafting, arthrodesis of the DIP joints in the setting of an intact FDS tendon, or tendon transfers. Treatment may be influenced by patient factors, such as compliance, general health condition, or the presence of infection and by the time elapsed since initial repair. Ruptures occurring in the early postoperative period (within 4 weeks from initial repair) may be primarily repaired; however, if the rupture occurs more than 4 to 6 weeks after the original repair, tendon grafting or a staged tendon reconstruction may be the more appropriate management option,[37] as scar adhesions with collapse and stiffening of the sheath may make primary repair impossible.

Various studies have reported that immediate rerepair of zone 1 and 2 flexor tendon injuries can result in good or excellent results in just more than 60% of cases.[14,40,42,48] A more recent study specifically addressing the outcome after immediate rerepair of zone 1 and 2 primary flexor tendon repair ruptures, however, reported on achieving excellent or good results in just more than 50% of the fingers.[49] In particular, the little finger has posed problems in terms of poor functional outcome in the setting of rupture of the primary repair. As a result, experts have considered implementing a policy of absolutely no direct rerepair in the little finger. However, given the inconsistent anatomy of the FDS tendon in the little finger, this may not be an option.[50]

Problems encountered during rerepair are mostly related to the bulk of the rerepair; tendon edema and increasingly frayed tendon ends may present obstacles to free tendon gliding. Given the existing space restriction, a single tendon repair has been proposed as potentially being more appropriate after a double tendon rupture along with resection of the FDS tendon to prevent adhesion formation under the A2 pulley.[49] Recently, the concept of combining stronger core sutures, pulley venting, and safer rehabilitation has been discussed.[51]

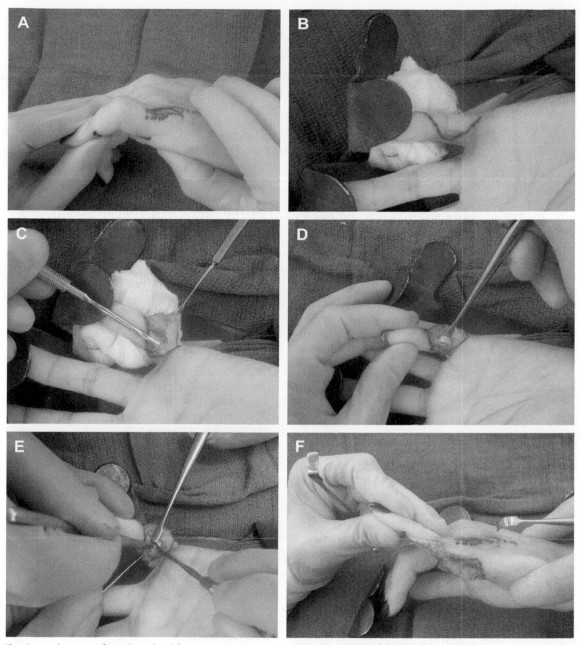

Fig. 2. Authors' preferred method for contracture release. (*A*) Preoperative image demonstrating limited passive extension secondary to PIP joint contracture. (*B*) Exposure is gained via Bruner zigzag incisions. (*C*) Flexor tenolysis is performed with blunt dissectors introduced into the tendon sheath. (*D*) Full release of the flexor tendon. (*E*) Release of the volar plate and checkrein ligaments. (*F*) Full passive extension after release.

Authors' Preferred Method

The authors recommend reexploration at the earliest suspicion of rupture. To recognize and address ruptures in a timely manner, close communication with a physical/hand therapist is critical. Exploration should be performed within 48 to 72 hours after the presumed rupture. Within this time frame, it is typically still possible to readvance the tendon and perform a primary repair. Should readvancement of the tendons not be possible, a staged tendon reconstruction is indicated. In the setting of an isolated FDS rupture with the FDP tendon being intact, it may be prudent to avoid the FDS repair because it may result in increased adhesion formation.

Wide exposure using Bruner zigzag incisions is recommended for staged tendon reconstruction. The distal end of the FDP tendon in zone 1 is isolated, the A2 and A4 pulleys are preserved, and any remaining FDS and FDP tendons are excised. A Hunter silicone rod is subsequently sutured to the distal tendon stump and passed through the preserved pulleys into the distal forearm. Postoperatively, the patient should undergo immediate physical therapy with passive ROM exercises to maintain full flexion and extension. Wound care is critical during this time period, as any degree of wound breakdown may result in infection of the silicone rod, which then requires removal. Any attempt of reinserting a Hunter rod has to wait until no signs of infection are present and soft tissue equilibrium is reached.

After 2 to 6 months, the second stage may be performed using tendon grafts (palmaris longus, plantaris, or long toe extensors). The authors recommend the use of long toe extensors from the second and third toes, as these are typically a good size match for the FDP tendons. The palmaris longus tendon is often too short to span from the distal phalanx to the forearm, and the plantaris is frequently too thin to allow for adequate function. Intrasynovial tendon grafts are increasingly being proposed, as theoretical advantages exist over extrasynovial tendon grafts. However, comparative clinical trials are lacking, and the case series present in the literature involve only a small number of patients, at times, with various injuries that further confound the functional outcome. Thus, based on the level of evidence present, one cannot strongly recommend intrasynovial tendon grafts over the time-honored extrasynovial grafts. In fact, a recent experimental study demonstrated superior tensile properties of extrasynovial tendons.[52–54]

Once the tendon graft is harvested, the Hunter rod is exposed proximally and distally. The tendon graft is sutured to the proximal end of the silicone rod, which is then removed distally, thus placing the tendon graft within the pseudosheath as the rod is withdrawn (**Fig. 3**). Distally, the tendon graft is sutured to the distal FDP tendon remnant (if >1 cm of tendon remains) or anchored to the bone via a suture anchor. Alternatively, the tendon graft can be secured to the bone, using the Bunnell pullout technique.

Proximally, an adequate motor muscle is identified. The authors prefer an adjoining FDP tendon. An FDS tendon may also be used. The proximal juncture is performed using the Pulvertaft weave technique. Postoperatively, the patient should undergo an early active motion protocol, however, with a slower progression.

PULLEY FAILURE/BOWSTRINGING

The pulley system is composed of 5 annular (A1–A5) and 3 cruciate pulleys (C1–C3). The alignment of these pulleys maintains the flexor tendons close to the joint's axis of rotation, converting tendon excursion into angular joint displacement. The A2 and A4 pulleys are widely accepted as being the most essential and responsible for preserving digital motion and strength.[55,56] Tang,[51] however, has demonstrated that excision of the A4 pulley does not entail adverse effects on function. Failure of the pulley system, as a result of direct trauma or careless surgical dissection, results in bowstringing with subsequent decrease in the ROM of the affected digit.[57,58]

Pulley failure typically results in delayed presentation of a patient because full finger flexion and extension are possible initially. Bowstringing invariably ensues after significant pulley insufficiency, which eventually results in progressive flexion contractures of the MCP, PIP, and DIP joints.[59] Diagnosis can be made clinically and by ultrasonography and magnetic resonance imaging.[60,61] Functional impairment of the pulley system can be prevented during flexor tendon repair by meticulous surgical technique, minimal manipulation of the annular pulleys and tendon repair through cruciate pulley windows, and preservation of as much of the uninjured pulley system and sheath as possible.[37]

Despite all efforts, pulley failure may still be encountered after flexor tendon repair. Reconstruction of the intricate pulley system is certainly among the most challenging tasks in hand surgery and rarely yields results equivalent to the preinjury state. The literature is replete with techniques for pulley reconstruction. However, 5 main types of pulley reconstruction represent the basis for the various modifications described in the literature. Contrary to the number of techniques proposed, clinical outcome data are extremely limited, making the decision to recommend a particular method difficult.[62]

Authors' Preferred Method

The authors prefer using tendon for pulley reconstruction. Donor tendons include the palmaris longus, partial flexor carpi radialis, or remnants of the FDS tendon. Depending on the intraoperative findings, the harvested tendon is either secured to the periosteum of the phalanx or wrapped circumferentially around the phalanx. Preservation of the neurovascular bundles is critical as is avoidance of any disruption of the extensor mechanism when attempting circumferential placement of the tendon graft.

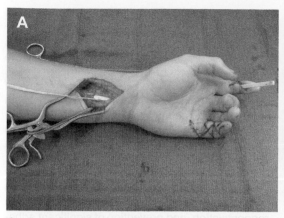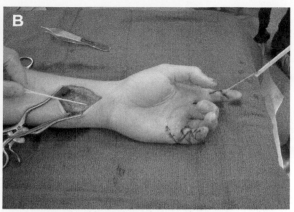

Fig. 3. Authors' preferred method for staged tendon grafting. (*A*) After proximal and distal exposure of the Hunter rod, the tendon graft is sutured to the proximal end of the silicone rod. (*B*) The tendon graft is subsequently placed within the pseudosheath as the silicone rod is withdrawn distally.

In cases of delayed flexor tendon repair, the occurrence of significant bowstringing is rare because scar formation prevents its progression. Again, wide exploration should be performed under local anesthesia to allow for active patient participation intraoperatively. If bowstringing is indeed observed, pulley reconstruction is performed as outlined earlier.

In general, the entire width of the native pulley does not need to be reconstructed. Furthermore, a period of immobilization postoperatively is certainly warranted to prevent secondary pulley failure. Immobilization will invariably lead to adhesion formation, and close follow-up is mandatory to avoid entering the cycle of reconstruction, immobilization, tenolysis, and physical therapy.

TRIGGERING

The most common cause of triggering is stenosing tenosynovitis. Trigger finger may also develop after flexor tendon injury. The 2 most common causes for development of trigger finger in this setting are either a bulky tendon repair or an unrecognized partial tendon laceration.

The repair site after a bulky tendon repair can catch on a pulley and contribute to triggering. Preventive measures include intraoperative assessment to identify areas that may interfere with unrestricted tendon gliding. Partial tendon sheath excision or pulley release may be indicated in this setting. These maneuvers should be performed cautiously, as bowstringing may result from excessive release. If triggering is encountered postoperatively after tendon healing is complete, different treatment modalities exist, including massage, ultrasound therapy, and steroid injections.[17] In select cases, reduction

tenoplasty may be considered. However, it is associated with an increased risk of tendon rupture.[63]

Partial tendon laceration is also a well-established cause of triggering.[64–67] Two mechanisms of triggering have been proposed for this occurrence: (1) a bulbous scar is formed at the area of laceration, with subsequent triggering as suggested by Kleinert[68]; (2) the edge of the lacerated tendon impinges at the entrance into the fibro-osseous retinacular system or at unrepaired portions of the sheath, with subsequent peeling away of tendon fibers from the site of injury, and the cut fibers fold on themselves and may create a nodule.[65,69]

The interval between initial trauma and development of triggering has been reported to range from 3 weeks up to 5 months.[70] In addition to triggering, symptoms may include localized tenderness at the site of previous injury along with a palpable swelling or nodular mass. The diagnosis is typically made based on history and clinical examination. Ultrasonography, however, may aid in diagnosis.[71]

Preventive measures to avoid triggering secondary to partial tendon laceration involve surgical exploration. Management of partial tendon lacerations is, however, controversial. Proponents of surgical repair of partial tendon lacerations report better results after suture and immobilization of partially severed tendons.[68,72] Others have reported excellent results without suturing, followed by early mobilization in partial tendon injuries involving up to 90% of the width of the tendon.[73–75]

Authors' Preferred Method

In the authors' opinion, triggering is a complication that is best treated by prevention. Aggressive exploration and repair of all cut ends is recommended to prevent scar formation originating from unrepaired cut ends. Despite an ongoing debate in the literature about suggested algorithms to perform a repair based on the percentage of tendon diameter cut, the authors feel that it is prudent to address even small lacerations with a 6-0 nonabsorbable monofilament suture. This suture is not intended to add significant strength to the tendon but rather to create a smooth epitendinous surface that allows unrestricted tendon gliding.

In the event of triggering postoperatively, early exploration is performed and any adhesions that may have formed are taken down. In most cases, the cut edges of the tendon will have already healed to some degree. Thus, direct repair of any triggering edges may not be feasible. In this case, partial venting of the pulleys is performed, which will resolve triggering while still preventing the occurrence of bowstringing.

INFECTION

Infections after flexor tendon repair are rare, but they can occur in some situations.[76,77] The most common cause of an infection is a significant degree of contamination during the initial trauma. The likelihood of infection increases with injuries related to agricultural or maritime activities.[78,79] The risk of infection varies with the type of injury and is higher after replantation,[76] injuries with concomitant fractures,[80] bite wounds,[81–84] and crush injuries.[85] Diabetes may also increase the infection rate.

The presence of severe contamination or frank infection must be addressed before any surgical repairs to the tendon are performed. Superficial infections can be treated with antibiotics, debridement, and irrigation. It is important to mention that prophylactic perioperative antibiotics have not been shown to decrease the incidence of infection in simple open flexor tendon injuries when thorough preoperative and perioperative wound care is performed.[86] Copious wound irrigation and debridement are therefore the most important steps in preventing infection. With deeper infections, drainage and antibiotics are typically indicated.

QUADRIGA

The quadriga phenomenon, also known as profundus blockage, was initially described by Bunnell and termed "quadriga" by Verdan.[87,88] It is caused by functional shortening of the FDP tendon of any of the 3 ulnar fingers. This may be the result of adhesions, joint contractures, or insertion of a short tendon graft. The anatomical basis for this phenomenon is the fact that the FDP tendons to the middle, ring, and small fingers share a common muscle belly. Hence, restricted flexion of one of these digits prevents full contraction of the shared ulnar belly of the FDP muscle with resultant restricted finger flexion in the remaining uninjured digits. Presenting symptoms include loss of flexion in the uninjured digits along with weakness of grip, particularly for small objects.[89]

This phenomenon may be prevented by proper tendon tensioning during primary repair, insertion of tendon grafts of adequate length during tendon reconstruction, and prevention of significant adhesion and joint contracture formation through meticulous surgical technique and appropriate postoperative rehabilitation. Treatment of quadriga when it occurs is directed toward the cause and hence is variable. It may include tenolysis, tendon lengthening, or even transection of the offending tendon to release the uninjured profundi and result in functional improvement.[17] When embarking on the surgical management of this rare complication, the authors recommend performing wide exploration under local anesthesia to allow patient participation.

LUMBRICAL PLUS DEFORMITY

The lumbrical muscles arise from the FDP tendons in the palm and insert distally into the dorsal extensor apparatus via the lateral bands. Normally, PIP and DIP joint flexion occurs in conjunction with simultaneous relaxation of the lumbrical muscles. Hence, the main function of the lumbrical muscles is coordination and control of delicate movement of the fingers.

The lumbrical plus deformity is the "paradoxical extension" of the interphalangeal joints when the patient attempts full flexion.[90,91] Paradoxical extension is the result of an FDP tendon that is functionally too long or is not present at all. Clinical scenarios that can cause this phenomenon are transection of the FDP tendon distal to the lumbrical origin, avulsion of the FDP insertion, an overlong flexor tendon graft, and amputation through the middle phalanx.[90–92] As a result, the force when attempting full flexion is transmitted to the extensor mechanism via the lumbricals and lateral bands before full flexion is reached.

Surgical treatment is aimed at restoring normal functional length of the FDP. Options include lumbrical muscle release, which may be performed under local anesthesia with minimal patient morbidity. Immediate functional improvement can be observed after this procedure.[90]

Alternatively, if the lumbrical plus deformity is caused by a tendon graft that is too long, placement of a graft of adequate length is indicated. Parkes[91] proposed to prophylactically divide the lumbrical muscle when inserting a flexor tendon graft to prevent paradoxical extension should the graft be a little too long. Again, principles of treatment include wide exploration under local anesthesia.

SUMMARY

The complexity of flexor tendon injury and repair is commonly underestimated by surgeons and patients. The incidence of the complications outlined in this article is best reduced by strict adherence to well-established principles of tendon repair and postoperative rehabilitation programs on initial treatment. Once complications are encountered, the surgeon must inform the patient that even in the best of hands, return to normal function may not be possible.

REFERENCES

1. Mass DP, Phillips CS. Preface - flexor tendon injuries. Hand Clin 2005;21(2):xi–xii.
2. Bunnell S. Repair of tendons in the fingers and description of two new instruments. Surg Gynecol Obstet 1918;26:103–10.
3. Beredjiklian PK. Biologic aspects of flexor tendon laceration and repair. J Bone Joint Surg Am 2003; 85:539–50.
4. Wade PJ, Muir IF, Hutcheon LL. Primary flexor tendon repair: the mechanical limitations of the modified Kessler technique. J Hand Surg Br 1986; 11(1):71–6.
5. Lee H. Double loop locking suture: a technique of tendon repair for early active mobilization. Part II: clinical experience. J Hand Surg Am 1990;15(6): 953–8.
6. Lister GD, Kleinert HE, Kutz JE, et al. Primary flexor tendon repair followed by immediate controlled mobilization. J Hand Surg Am 1977;2(6):441–51.
7. Chow JA, Thomes LJ, Dovelle S, et al. A combined regimen of controlled motion following flexor tendon repair in "no man's land". Plast Reconstr Surg 1987; 79(3):447–55.
8. Bainbridge LC, Robertson C, Gillies D, et al. A comparison of post-operative mobilization of flexor tendon repairs with "passive flexion-active extension" and "controlled active motion" techniques. J Hand Surg Br 1994;19(4):517–21.
9. Duran RJ, House RG. Controlled passive motion following tendon repairs in zone 2 and 3. In: American academy of orthopedic surgeons: symposium on tendon surgery in the hand. St. Louis (MO): CV Mosby Co; 1975. p. 105–14.
10. Strickland JW. Development of flexor tendon surgery: twenty-five years of progress. J Hand Surg Am 2000;25(2):214–35.
11. Thien TB, Becker JH, Theis JC. Rehabilitation after flexor tendon injuries in the hand. Cochrane Database Syst Rev 2004;(4):CD003979.
12. Karlander LE, Berggren M, Larsson M, et al. Improved results in zone 2 flexor tendon injuries with a modified technique of immediate controlled mobilization. J Hand Surg Br 1993;18:26–30.
13. Chan TK, Ho CO, Lee WK, et al. Functional outcome of the hand following flexor tendon repair at the 'no man's land'. J Orthop Surg (Hong Kong) 2006; 14(2):178–83.
14. Small JO, Brennen MD, Colville J. Early active mobilisation following flexor tendon repair in zone 2. J Hand Surg Br 1989;14(4):383–91.
15. Kitsis CK, Wade PJ, Krikler SJ, et al. Controlled active motion following primary flexor tendon repair: a prospective study over 9 years. J Hand Surg Br 1998;23(3):344–9.
16. O'Connell SJ, Moore MM, Strickland JW, et al. Results of zone I and zone II flexor tendon repairs in children. J Hand Surg Am 1994;19(1):48–52.
17. Taras JS, Gray RM, Culp RW. Complications of flexor tendon injuries. Hand Clin 1994;10(1):93–109.
18. Lister G. Pitfalls and complications of flexor tendon surgery. Hand Clin 1985;1:133–46.
19. Strickland JW. The scientific basis for advances in flexor tendon surgery. J Hand Ther 2005;18(2): 94–110.
20. Potenza AD. Critical evaluation of flexor-tendon healing and adhesion formation within artificial digital sheaths. J Bone Joint Surg Am 1963;45:1217–33.
21. Chow SP, Pun WK, So YC, et al. A prospective study of 245 open digital fractures of the hand. J Hand Surg Br 1991;16(2):137–40.
22. Gelberman RH, Vandeberg JS, Manske PR, et al. The early stages of flexor tendon healing: a morphologic study of the first fourteen days. J Hand Surg Am 1985;10(6 Pt 1):776–84.
23. Zhao C, Amadio PC, Zobitz ME, et al. Gliding characteristics of tendon repair in canine flexor digitorum profundus tendons. J Orthop Res 2001; 19(4):580–6.
24. Stein T, Ali A, Hamman J, et al. A randomized biomechanical study of zone II human flexor tendon repairs analyzed in an in vitro model. J Hand Surg Am 1998;23(6):1046–51.
25. Feehan LM, Beauchene JG. Early tensile properties of healing chicken flexor tendons: early controlled passive motion versus postoperative immobilization. J Hand Surg Am 1990;15(1):63–8.
26. Khanna A, Friel M, Gougoulias N, et al. Prevention of adhesions in surgery of the flexor tendons of the

hand: what is the evidence? Br Med Bull 2009;90: 85–109.

27. Strickland JW. Flexor tendon surgery. Part 2: free tendon grafts and tenolysis. J Hand Surg Br 1989; 14(4):368–82.

28. Strickland JW. Flexor tenolysis. Hand Clin 1985;1(1): 121–32.

29. Boyer MI, Strickland JW, Engles D, et al. Flexor tendon repair and rehabilitation: state of the art in 2002. Instr Course Lect 2003;52:137–61.

30. Schneider LH. Tenolysis and capsulectomy after hand fractures. Clin Orthop Relat Res 1996;327:72–8.

31. Foucher G, Lenoble E, Ben Youssef K, et al. A postoperative regime after digital flexor tenolysis. A series of 72 patients. J Hand Surg Br 1993;18(1): 35–40.

32. Hahn P, Krimmer H, Müller L, et al. Outcomes of flexor tenolysis after injury in zone 2. Handchir Mikrochir Plast Chir 1996;28(4):198–203.

33. Eggli S, Dietsche A, Eggli S, et al. Tenolysis after combined digital injuries in zone II. Ann Plast Surg 2005;55(3):266–71.

34. Feldscher SB. Flexor tenolysis. Hand Surg 2002; 7(1):61–74.

35. Bruner JM. The zig-zag volar-digital incision for flexor-tendon surgery. Plast Reconstr Surg 1967; 40(6):571–4.

36. Tang JB. Clinical outcomes with flexor tendon repair. Hand Clin 2005;21:199–210.

37. Lilly SI, Messer TM. Complications after treatment of flexor tendon injuries. J Am Acad Orthop Surg 2006; 14(7):387–96.

38. Tang JB, Shi D, Gu YQ, et al. Double and multiple looped suture tendon repair. J Hand Surg Br 1994; 19(6):699–703.

39. Baktir A, Türk CY, Kabak S, et al. Flexor tendon repair in zone II followed by early active mobilization. J Hand Surg Br 1996;21(5):624–8.

40. Harris SB, Harris D, Foster AJ, et al. The aetiology of acute rupture of flexor tendon repairs in zones 1 and 2 of the fingers during early mobilization. J Hand Surg Br 1999;24(3):275–80.

41. Golash A, Kay A, Warner JG, et al. Efficacy of AD-CON-T/N after primary tendon repair in Zone II: a controlled clinical trial. J Hand Surg Br 2003; 28(2):113–5.

42. Elliot D, Moiemen NS, Flemming AF, et al. The rupture rate of acute flexor tendon repairs mobilized by the controlled active motion regimen. J Hand Surg Br 1994;19(5):607–12.

43. Zhao C, Moran SL, Cha SS, et al. An analysis of factors associated with failure of tendon repair in the canine model. J Hand Surg Am 2007;32(4): 518–25.

44. Tang JB, Xu Y, Wang B. Repair strength of tendons of varying gliding curvature: a study in a curvilinear model. J Hand Surg Am 2003;28(2):243–9.

45. Peck FH, Kennedy SM, Watson JS, et al. An evaluation of the influence of practitioner-led Hand Clin on rupture rates following primary tendon repair in the hand. Br J Plast Surg 2004;57(1):45–9.

46. Zhao C, Amadio PC, Zobitz ME, et al. Effect of synergistic motion on flexor digitorum profundus tendon excursion. Clin Orthop Relat Res 2002;396:223–30.

47. Leddy JP. Flexor tendons—acute injuries. In: Green DP, editor. Operative hand surgery. New York: Churchill Livingstone; 1982. p. 1359.

48. Allen BN, Frykman GK, Unsell RS, et al. Ruptured flexor tendon tenorrhaphies in zone 2: repair and rehabilitation. J Hand Surg Am 1987;12(1):18–21.

49. Dowd MB, Figus A, Harris SB, et al. The results of immediate re-repair of zone 1 and 2 primary flexor tendon repairs which rupture. J Hand Surg Br 2006;31(5):507–13.

50. Elliot D, Barbieri CH, Evans RB, et al. IFSSH flexor tendon committee report 2007. J Hand Surg Eur Vol 2007;32(3):346–56.

51. Tang JB. Indications, methods, postoperative motion and outcome evaluation of primary flexor tendon repairs in Zone 2. J Hand Surg Eur Vol 2007;32(2):118–29.

52. Leversedge FJ, Zelouf D, Williams C, et al. Flexor tendon grafting to the hand: an assessment of the intrasynovial donor-tendon – A preliminary single-cohort study. J Hand Surg Am 2000;25(4):721–30.

53. Beris AE, Darlis NA, Korompilas AV, et al. Two-stage flexor tendon reconstruction in zone II using a silicone rod and a pedicled intrasynovial graft. J Hand Surg Am 2003;28(4):652–60.

54. Shin RH, Zhao C, Zobitz ME, et al. Mechanical properties of intrasynovial and extrasynovial tendon fascicles. Clin Biomech (Bristol, Avon) 2008;23(2): 236–41.

55. Doyle JR. Anatomy of the flexor tendon sheath and pulley system: a current review. J Hand Surg Am 1989;14:349–51.

56. Barton NJ. Experimental study of optimal location of flexor tendon pulleys. Plast Reconstr Surg 1969; 43(2):125–9.

57. Bowers WH, Kuzma GR, Bynum DK. Closed traumatic rupture of finger flexor pulleys. J Hand Surg Am 1985;10(5):620–2.

58. Bollen SR. Injury to the A2 pulley in rock climbers. J Hand Surg Br 1990;15(2):268–70.

59. Naidu SH, Rinkus K. Multiple-loop, uniform-tension flexor pulley reconstruction. J Hand Surg Am 2007; 32(2):265–8.

60. Klauser A, Frauscher F, Bodner G, et al. Finger pulley injuries in extreme rock climbers: depiction with dynamic US. Radiology 2002;222(3):755–61.

61. Bodner G, Rudisch A, Gabl M, et al. Diagnosis of digital flexion tendon annular pulley disruption: comparison of high frequency ultrasound and MRI. Ultraschall Med 1999;20(4):131–6.

62. Mehta V, Phillips CS. Flexor tendon pulley reconstruction. Hand Clin 2005;21(2):245–51.
63. Serdage H, Kleinert HE. Reduction flexor tenoplasty. Treatment of stenosing flexor tenosynovitis distal to the first pulley. J Hand Surg Am 1981;6(6):543–4.
64. Janecki CJ Jr. Triggering of the finger caused by flexor-tendon laceration. J Bone Joint Surg Am 1976;58(8):1174–5.
65. Bilos ZJ, Hui PW, Stamelos S. Trigger finger following partial flexor tendon laceration. Hand 1977;9(3):232–3.
66. Schlenker JD, Lister GD, Kleinert HE. Three complications of untreated partial laceration of flexor tendon–entrapment, rupture, and triggering. J Hand Surg Am 1981;6(4):392–8.
67. Frewin PR, Scheker LR. Triggering secondary to an untreated partially-cut flexor tendon. J Hand Surg Br 1989;14(4):419–21.
68. Kleinert HE. Should an incompletely severed tendon be sutured? Commentary. Plast Reconstr Surg 1976; 57(2):236.
69. al-Qattan MM, Posnick JC, Lin KY. Triggering after partial tendon laceration. J Hand Surg Br 1993; 18(2):241–6.
70. Tohyama M, Tsujio T, Yanagida I. Trigger finger caused by an old partial flexor tendon laceration: a case report. Hand Surg 2005;10(1):105–8.
71. Fujiwara M. A case of trigger finger following partial laceration of flexor digitorum superficialis and review of the literature. Arch Orthop Trauma Surg 2005; 125(6):430–2.
72. Chow SP, Yu OD. An experimental study on incompletely cut chicken tendons–a comparison of two methods of management. J Hand Surg Br 1984; 9(2):121–5.
73. Wray RC Jr, Holtman B, Weeks PM. Clinical treatment of partial tendon lacerations without suturing and with early motion. Plast Reconstr Surg 1977; 59(2):231–4.
74. Wray RC Jr, Weeks PM. Treatment of partial tendon lacerations. Hand 1980;12(2):163–6.
75. al-Qattan MM. Conservative management of zone II partial flexor tendon lacerations greater than half the width of the tendon. J Hand Surg Am 2000;25(6): 1118–21.
76. Maloon S, de V de Beer J, Opitz M, et al. Acute flexor tendon sheath infections. J Hand Surg Am 1990;15:3.
77. Schneider LH. Complications in tendon injury and surgery. Hand Clin 1986;2:2.
78. Reginato AJ, Feneiro JL, O'Connor CR, et al. Clinical and penetrating foreign body injury to the joints, bursae, and tendon sheaths. Arthritis Rheum 1990; 33:12.
79. Hudson DA, De Chalain TM. Hand infections secondary to fish bone injuries. Ann R Coll Surg Engl 1994;76(2):99–101.
80. Sloan JP, Dove AF, Maheson M, et al. Antibiotics in open fractures of the distal phalanx? J Hand Surg Br 1987;12:123–4.
81. Nunley DL, Sasaki T, Atkins A, et al. Hand infections in hospitalized patients. Am J Surg 1980; 140:374–6.
82. Glass KD. Factors related to the resolution of treated hand infections. J Hand Surg 1982;7: 388–94.
83. Dellinger EP, Wertz MJ, Miller Sd, et al. Hand infections: bacteriology and treatment: a prospective study. Arch Surg 1988;123:745–50.
84. Dunbar JF. Serious infections following wounds and bites of the hand. N Z Med J 1988;101:368–9.
85. Fitzgerald RH, Cooney WP, Washington JA, et al. Bacterial colonization of mutilating hand injuries and its treatment. J Hand Surg 1977;2:85–9.
86. Stone JF, Davidson JSD. The role of antibiotics and timing of repair in flexor tendon injuries of the hand. Ann Plast Surg 1998;40:7–13.
87. Bunnell S. Reconstructive surgery of the hand. Surg Gynecol Obstet 1924;34:259–74.
88. Verdan C. Syndrome of the quadriga. Surg Clin North Am 1960;40:425–6.
89. Horton TC, Sauerland S, Davis TR. The effect of flexor digitorum profundus quadriga on grip strength. J Hand Surg Eur Vol 2007;32(2):130–4.
90. Parkes A. The "lumbrical plus" finger. Hand 1970; 2(2):164–5.
91. Parkes A. The "lumbrical plus" finger. J Bone Joint Surg Br 1971;53(2):236–9.
92. Goodwin DR, Salama R. Lumbrical plus finger. Injury 1981;13(1):82–3.

The Stiff Finger

F. Thomas D. Kaplan, MD

KEYWORDS

- Finger • Contracture • Stiffness
- Proximal interphalangeal joint
- Metacarpophalangeal joint • Tendon adhesions

The stiff finger is a frequently encountered entity in hand surgical practice. It stems from a myriad of causes, may have multiple components, and requires a variety of solutions. Simple stiff fingers may result from a minor proximal interphalangeal (PIP) joint sprain in which the patient overprotects and self-limits motion, whereas a patient with a table saw injury requiring bone, tendon, and nerve repair presents a more complex problem. A true understanding of the ideal treatments for the stiff finger requires a basic understanding of the local milieu that arises from injury and the anatomic features that are at risk for pathologic changes. Hand surgeons must be able to help patients understand the various factors at play and the time course of wound healing and injury-induced inflammation, because an educated and motivated patient is the best ally in the battle against the stiff finger.

BIOLOGY OF WOUND HEALING

After a traumatic event, infection, or surgical insult, a predictable series of events is set into motion. The magnitude of the response and the duration depends on multiple factors. Local tissue injury triggers the onset of the healing response, which is comprised of three phases: (1) inflammatory, (2) tissue-producing, and (3) tissue remodeling. These phases overlap in time, and the ongoing events in each phase determine the elements that contribute to finger stiffness, and the opportunities available to mitigate those factors.

Beginning with initial injury and tissue disruption, vasoactive and chemotactic factors are produced by injured parenchymal cells and the activated coagulation and complement pathways.[1] The inflammatory cascade results in increased capillary permeability, which allows protein-rich exudate to leak out into the interstitial space. There is also a decreased ability to transport the fluid back out by way of lymphatics, resulting in edema. This extracellular exudative fluid contributes to the stiff finger through an increased resistance to movement, joint capsular distention, and swelling of the articular capsule and ligaments.[2] The exudates also contain fibrinogen, which can turn into fibrin, leading to interstitial scar.[3]

The chemotactic factors produced by injured cells and activated platelets recruit inflammatory leukocytes to the site of injury. These monocytes, neutrophils, and macrophages act to remove foreign debris and necrotic tissue from the wound and secrete matrix metalloproteinases (including collagenase) clearing the injured area and creating the void that is filled by scar tissue.[4] Approximately 4 days after injury new stroma (granulation tissue) begins to fill the void as fibroblasts proliferate and migrate into the wound. New capillaries form and invade the wound by angiogenesis, while macrophages continue to aid in remodeling.

Once the wound has closed and the dermis healed, wound contracture ceases, but scar contraction may continue. Collagen cross-linking both within and between tissues promotes adhesion formation and joint stiffness.[5] The interstitial scar attaches to, and becomes part of, the normal tissues it is in contact with, obliterating normal tissue planes. Fibroblasts differentiate into myofibroblasts, which are the cells primarily responsible for scar contracture.[3] The net result is a wound in which normal gliding structures have more resistance to motion, and are surrounded by exudate and interstitial scar, which connects them to adjacent, nonmobile structures.

EARLY INTERVENTIONS

In the early stages of injury, stiffness can be limited and corrected with appropriate management. The

Indiana Hand to Shoulder Center, 8501 Harcourt Road, Indianapolis, IN 46260, USA
E-mail address: tdk@hand.md

Hand Clin 26 (2010) 191–204
doi:10.1016/j.hcl.2010.02.001

hand.theclinics.com

factors that lead to stiff fingers, including edema, pain, immobilization, and patient participation, should be assessed and appropriate interventions begun. Often, patients come to the office after injury poorly splinted and poorly educated on edema control. The first step is to identify the patient's injury and decide the appropriate treatment. It is then known what needs to be immobilized, what can move, and what may need surgical treatment, planning treatment not only on the injury, but also the patient's entire arm. For example, patients presenting with a distal radius fracture often keep their arms in a sling. They allow their fingers to become swollen, and do not move their shoulder, elbow, or fingers well. What results is all too familiar: not only does the patient have a wrist that needs therapy, but they must also work out their frozen shoulder and stiff hand, decreasing the amount of time they are able to spend on their wrist.

The educated patient is a strong ally. Once the treatment for the injury has been determined, the clinician then needs to ensure the patient understands the plan and what their role is to promote optimal healing. This begins with aggressive edema control including elevation and compressive dressings. Patients should be taught to keep the hand higher than heart level until the swelling has resolved. Early motion can also help control swelling, while limiting stiffness. Joints not needing protection should not be blocked by the splint or cast, and should be kept moving through their full range of motion using both active and passive modalities.

Treatment of the injured area can either set the stage for an excellent outcome or provide a recipe for disaster. Fracture malunion can lead to tendon imbalance, alteration of joint biomechanics, and bony obstruction to motion. Fracture stabilization may allow early motion (rigid fixation); preclude motion (poor construct strength, persistent instability); allow protected partial motion (dorsal block k-wire); and promote tendon adhesions (bulk and location of implants, piercing of tendons with k-wires, transarticular fixation). Tendon and ligament repair may allow full or partial arc active motion, passive motion, or necessitate immobilization. Ideal treatment optimizes fracture stability, tendon and ligament repair strength, and restoration of the soft tissue envelope.

Following the initial phases of protected motion, and once the injured and repaired structures have gained sufficient structural integrity, rehabilitation can advance. In patients with simple injuries, often the progression to full active and passive motion followed by strengthening is all that is necessary to regain normal function. In patients with more complex injuries, and those showing a tendency toward development of a stiff finger, more aggressive interventions are required. This typically involves the use of dynamic or static-progressive splinting to restore the soft tissues back to their normal lengths and elasticity. The goal is to restore a supple finger with full passive motion. Limited active motion can then be addressed surgically if necessary.

LATE TREATMENT

Once the inflammatory cascade has ended, the soft tissues reach equilibrium. This point varies in each patient and may occur within the first 2 to 3 months, or may take up to 6 months. Patients at this point have frequently reached a plateau in their range of motion, no longer having fluctuating edema, and timing is now appropriate to assess their finger for further surgical intervention. The surgeon should keep in mind the motivation the patient exhibited during the early stages of healing, in addition to the objective findings, when determining the appropriateness of a surgical procedure. On physical examination, the hand and fingers should have minimal or no edema or induration. Scars should be mature and hypersensitivity absent. Each joint should be carefully measured for both active and passive range of motion. Note should be made if measurements are limited by patient pain or effort. The presence of obvious deformity may alert the clinician to an underlying tendon imbalance, malunion, or nonunion.

The pathology responsible for the stiff finger can now be determined. It may be caused by tendon adhesions, myotendonous contracture, joint capsular contracture, arthrofibrosis, or a combination of these. Underlying causes, such as malunion, nonunion, or a poor soft tissue envelope, should be excluded or treated first if present. The treatment must be tailored to the pathology, and the clinician must be systematic in designing not only the appropriate procedures, but also the best sequence of procedures. A classification system based on six possible combinations of limited active or passive motion was described by Jupiter and colleagues[6] in 2007. I have added two additional categories, Type 7 and Type 8, to complete the system such that all possible combinations of limited motion are included (**Table 1**). By determining the appropriate category into which the patient's finger falls, one can better understand the pathologic structures that are responsible for the stiffness, and design appropriate treatment.

Table 1
Stiff finger classification

	Motion Loss	Dorsal Disease	Palmar Disease	Possible Associated Conditions	Treatment
Type 1	Limited passive flexion Limited passive extension	Extensor adhesions Dorsal capsuloligamentous contracture	A2 pulley insufficiency Palmar plate contracture Accessory collateral contracture Skin deficiency	Flexor tendon adhesions Flexor tendon disruption	Stage 1 Extensor tenolysis Dorsal capsulectomy Flexor check Stage 2 Flexor tenolysis, reconstruction Palmar plate, checkrein release
Type 2	Limited passive flexion Limited active extension	Extensor adhesions Dorsal capsuloligamentous contracture		Flexor tendon adhesions Flexor tendon disruption	Stage 1 Extensor tenolysis Dorsal capsulectomy Flexor check Stage 2 Flexor tenolysis, reconstruction
Type 3	Limited active flexion Limited passive extension		Flexor tendon adhesions Flexor tendon disruption A2 pulley insufficiency Palmar plate contracture Accessory collateral contracture Skin deficiency		Flexor tenolysis Flexor tendon reconstruction Pulley reconstruction Palmar plate, checkrein release Accessory collateral ligament release Skin contracture release, resurfacing
Type 4	Limited active flexion Limited active extension	Extensor subluxation Excessive length of extensor tendon	Flexor tendon adhesions Flexor tendon disruption		Stage 1 Extensor rebalancing, reconstruction Stage 2 Flexor tendon tenolysis, reconstruction
Type 5	Limited passive extension		Palmar plate contracture Accessory collateral contracture Palmar fibromatosis Palmar skin contracture		Palmar plate, checkrein release Accessory collateral ligament release Fasciectomy Skin contracture release, resurfacing
Type 6	Limited active flexion		Flexor tendon adhesions Flexor tendon disruption		Flexor tenolysis Flexor tendon reconstruction
Type 7	Limited passive flexion	Scar, burn contracture	Bone block (eg, retrocondylar fossa)		Skin contracture release, resurfacing Excision of bony block
Type 8	Limited active extension	Extensor disruption (central slip, terminal tendon rupture)			Splinting Extensor tendon repair, reconstruction

The Type 1 finger lacks passive flexion and passive extension. This implicates both palmar and dorsal disease. The lack of passive flexion signifies dorsal capsular contracture, often accompanied by extensor tendon adhesions. Limited passive extension is caused by palmar disease, and may have one or multiple causes, including palmar plate and collateral ligament contracture, skin contracture, and pulley incompetence. Flexor tendon adhesions also are often present, but cannot be assessed clinically because of the loss of full passive flexion.

Treatment of the Type 1 finger begins with ensuring an adequate attempt has been made to regain passive mobility through aggressive hand therapy. I have found it helpful to outline clearly to the patient the number of structures that are diseased. For a Type 1 finger with limited PIP joint motion, I tell the patient the joint itself is stiff, like a rusted door hinge. The tendons that straighten and bend the finger are also likely caught up in scar, but freeing up the tendons does not do any good until the hinge is free and can be moved. By regaining the passive motion of the joint, one can reduce the number of surgeries necessary and also improve the ultimate outcome. For example, in the patient with Type 1 stiffness following flexor tendon repair, they have dorsal and palmar stiffness of the joint, and probable flexor tendon adhesions. The extensor tendon system is likely not adhered. Treatment requires two stages: first to regain full passive flexion of the finger, and then to address the palmar side with capsular release and possible flexor tenolysis. Surgery on both the palmar and dorsal sides of the finger is almost never performed at the same time. This degree of surgical insult leads to increased postoperative swelling, pain, and the risk for marginal wound necrosis. The net effect is often significant recurrent scar formation, contracture, and compromised gain in motion.

Additionally, it is important to maximize the gains obtained from the first procedure, and allow the soft tissues to regain equilibrium, before the second procedure. Surgery on a finger with persistent edema, indurated tissues, and immature scar often leads to compromised results. A minimum of 3 months,[7] and up to 6 to 9 months,[8] has been advocated as the appropriate amount of time to wait between surgeries. Once the patient understands that by regaining their passive flexion through therapy they require one less surgery, and eliminate a 6-month recovery phase, they often become a more active participant in their treatment putting forth the effort needed for optimal results. This also lets patients decide whether further surgery is worthwhile to them,

allowing them to make an informed decision for surgical reconstruction.

THERAPY FOR THE STIFF FINGER

The first step in treatment of an established finger contracture is with a therapy program geared to stretching scar. The patient should have already been instructed in, and been compliant with, standard active, active-assisted, and passive range-of-motion exercises. When these have failed to restore full mobility, techniques that are more effective in elongating tissue are needed. Fortunately, significant improvements in motion can often be achieved with the addition of dynamic and static-progressive splinting.

Dynamic splinting is the use of traction devices, such as rubber bands, to alter the range of passive motion of a joint.[9] They are optimally worn for extended periods of time, up to 8 to 12 hours, for each session. Through prolonged, constant load, tissues respond by plastic deformation. By definition, this deformation is permanent, in that after removal of the load, the tissue remains in its' elongated state. This is in contrast to elastic deformation, which occurs with rapid loading, and results only in temporary tissue elongation. Dynamic splinting produces plastic deformation through creep. Creep is the deformation of tissue that occurs while placed under constant stress for an extended period of time. If the tissue is unloaded before failure occurs, then the tissue remains permanently lengthened as a result of viscoplastic properties.

Static progressive splinting and serial casting also produce plastic deformation, although through a different process (stress relaxation). Stress relaxation occurs when a material is held at a constant deformation. The amount of force required to maintain the deformation decreases with time, as the tissue stretches by plastic deformation, until equilibrium is reached.

Both methods have been shown effective for improving motion in contracted joints.[10–13] Dynamic splints are readily available, because they can be made from materials present in most therapy offices. Their main disadvantage is the prolonged duration of wear necessary for lasting improvement, which may affect patient compliance. Static-progressive splints are well tolerated, effective, and require significantly less treatment time.[12] Regardless of the method used, it is critical to make the patient understand that unless they can feel the discomfort of the stretch, no gains can be expected. They continually need to adjust the tension on the splints while they are wearing them to maintain the sense of discomfort. If they do not, once the finger has loosened in the first 5 to 10 minutes of wear, further gains do not occur.

THERAPY FOR LIMITED PASSIVE FLEXION

My preference for restoration of passive flexion involves several modalities, including taping, interphalangeal slings, and dynamic flexion splinting. Taping is the first modality added to the stiff finger, and involves placing tape from the dorsum of the hand, along the extensor surface of the finger across the metacarpophalangeal and PIP joints to the palm and volar wrist (**Fig. 1**A). This holds the hand in a position of composite flexion, which stretches the dorsal capsules of the metacarpophalangeal and PIP joints. Patients are instructed to perform taping three to four times daily, maintaining the stretch for 20 minutes.

If there are limited gains with taping after 1 to 2 weeks, dynamic splinting or interphalangeal (IP) slings are added. Dynamic splints can be fashioned to place tension on both metacarpophalangeal and PIP joints, or by adding a proximal phalanx block (**Fig. 1**B), can maximize tension on the PIP joint. Patients are encouraged to use the splint continuously for 30 minutes, four to six times per day.

IP slings (**Fig. 1**C) are very effective for PIP and distal interphalangeal (DIP) joint stiffness, but can only be used once patients have regained approximately 30 to 40 degrees of PIP and DIP flexion.

Patients are instructed to wear them on the affected fingers four to six times daily for 15 to 20 minutes. Because they are small and portable, I find that patients have improved compliance, and are able to use them more frequently than they would a dynamic splint. It is also easy for them to adjust the tension themselves, cinching up the loop on the sling as IP flexion improves.

THERAPY FOR LIMITED PASSIVE EXTENSION

For the finger with a flexion contracture, I use dynamic and static-progressive methods. Initial attempts to stretch out joints with less than a 30-degree contracture begin with use of a spring finger extension-assist Lois M. Barber (LMB) splint (**Fig. 2**A) worn for 30 minutes at a time, six times daily. If the LMB split is not providing much gain, or does not fit the patient well, a Bunnell safety-pin splint is used (**Fig. 2**B). The safety-pin splint can provide a more forceful stretch than can the LMB splint, but is more difficult to take on and off. Patients are also fitted with a static extension splint holding the finger in their maximally extended position, which is worn while sleeping.

For digits with more severe contracture (> 30–35 degrees), and those not responsive to LMB and safety-pin splinting, dynamic extension splinting is indicated. The short dorsal outrigger is the typical splint used (**Fig. 2**C), and patients are instructed to use it four to six times per day for 30

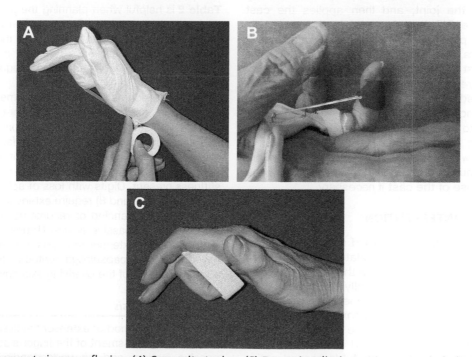

Fig. 1. Therapy to improve flexion. (*A*) Composite taping. (*B*) Dynamic splinting with proximal phalanx block to concentrate force on PIP joint. (*C*) IP slings stretching both PIP and DIP joints.

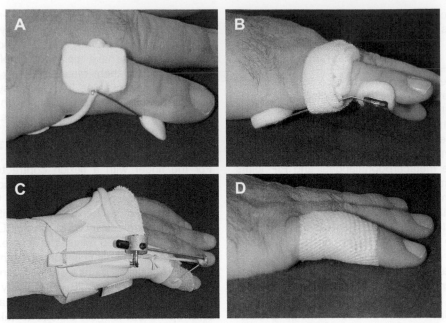

Fig. 2. Splints to improve extension. (*A*) LMB splint. (*B*) Bunnell safety-pin splint. (*C*) Short dorsal outrigger (dynamic extension splint). (*D*) Serial cast.

minutes. When all else has failed, for recalcitrant contractures, static-progressive stretching may be necessary. Serial casting can be incredibly effective for these stiff fingers (**Fig. 2**D). Patients must be compliant and able to visit the therapist every 2 to 3 days. The therapist first maximally stretches the joint, and then applies the cast around the PIP joint to maintain the maximally extended position. The patient then returns in 2 to 3 days, the joint is stretched further, and a new cast applied. The process is repeated until either there are no further gains, or full extension is achieved. At this point the cast can often be slid on and off the finger, and the patient is instructed to wean use of the cast removing it for increasing periods of time. During the period of weaning, while patients are regaining joint flexion, they are taught to recognize loss of extension, and increase use of the cast if necessary.

SURGICAL INTERVENTION

Once the patient has regained normal soft tissue equilibrium, and reached a plateau in their range of motion, one can proceed with surgical interventions, if still necessary. Ideally the patient with a Type 1 finger has now regained passive flexion, passive extension, or both, converting their finger to a Type 2 (decreased passive flexion and active extension); Type 3 (decreased active flexion and passive extension); or Type 4 (decreased active flexion and extension). In the process or working

out the joint contracture, patients often regain some improvement in their active motion, and a Type 1 finger can also become a Type 6 (decreased active flexion).

Procedures are staged when there is concomitant palmar and dorsal disease. The algorithm in **Table 2** is helpful when planning the procedures that may be necessary. One can then establish the overall treatment plan and educate the patient on the number of surgeries required, necessary therapy after surgery, and time required for maximal benefit.

Dorsal procedures are usually performed before palmar ones, and may include extensor tenolysis, dorsal capsulectomy, extensor reconstruction, and skin contracture release or resurfacing. The structures to be addressed are identified based on the nature of the original injury and the type of stiffness present. Digits with loss of active extension (Types 2, 4, and 8) require extensor tenolysis or extensor rebalancing or reconstruction. Digits with decreased passive flexion (Types 1, 2, and 7) require both extensor tenolysis and release of the dorsal joint capsuloligamentous structures, and assessment of the overlying skin envelope.

Extensor Tenolysis

My preferred method of extensor tenolysis begins with a clear assessment of the finger's active and passive motion, and an understanding of the possible root causes of the adhesions. For

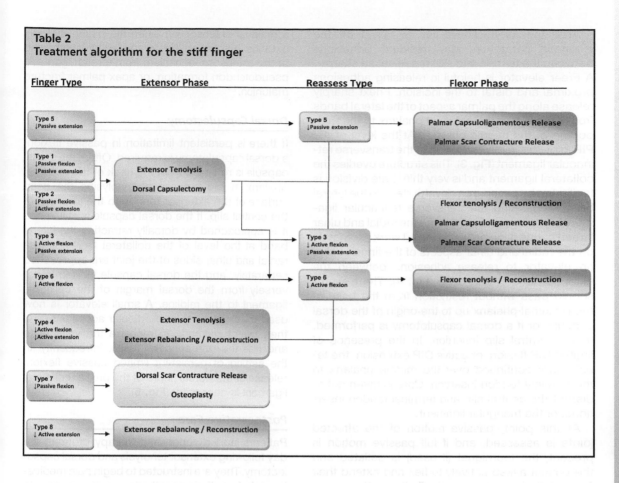

Table 2
Treatment algorithm for the stiff finger

Finger Type	Extensor Phase	Reassess Type	Flexor Phase
Type 5 ↓Passive extension		**Type 5** ↓Passive extension	**Palmar Capsuloligamentous Release** / **Palmar Scar Contracture Release**
Type 1 ↓Passive flexion ↓Passive extension	**Extensor Tenolysis** / **Dorsal Capsulectomy**		
Type 2 ↓Passive flexion ↓Active extension			**Flexor tenolysis / Reconstruction** / **Palmar Capsuloligamentous Release** / **Palmar Scar Contracture Release**
Type 3 ↓Active flexion ↓Passive extension		**Type 3** ↓Active flexion ↓Passive extension	
Type 6 ↓Active flexion		**Type 6** ↓Active flexion	**Flexor tenolysis / Reconstruction**
Type 4 ↓Active flexion ↓Active extension	**Extensor Tenolysis** / **Extensor Rebalancing / Reconstruction**		
Type 7 ↓Passive flexion	**Dorsal Scar Contracture Release** / **Osteoplasty**		
Type 8 ↓Active extension	**Extensor Rebalancing / Reconstruction**		

patients with adhesions after fracture, knowledge of the location of the fracture, residual malalignment, and hardware present is crucial for surgical planning. For instance, the patient with a minimally displaced proximal phalangeal neck fracture treated with cast immobilization may only have a very limited area of the tendon spot-welded to the bone, as opposed to the patient with a distal radius fracture whose finger has gotten stiff because of significant persistent edema and lack of motion whose entire digital extensor mechanism is adherent.

Surgery is performed under a local anesthetic with short-acting or no sedation. Tourniquet use is limited, or avoided with the use of digital block with epinephrine,[14] to preserve the patient's ability actively to move the digit intraoperatively. When a tourniquet is used, it is placed on the forearm, and use is limited to 20 to 30 minutes to avoid muscle paresis. Assessing the patients' active motion can result in the patient rupturing residual adhesions and ensures that their extensor lag has been eliminated. It can also improve patient motivation; by lowering the drapes and letting the patient see how far they are able to bend their finger, they gain a visual goal that helps them as they work through the swelling and pain in subsequent therapy.

The incision is centered over the area of most likely adhesions. In patients with adhesions following extensor tendon injury proximal to the finger, the tenolysis is first performed at the site of repair or transfer. Previous incisions may be used, and are extended proximally and distally into areas free of scar, allowing for the accurate definition of normal tissue planes. In the finger, I prefer a curvilinear incision over the dorsum of the finger, centered at the PIP joint. Dissection is performed with loupe magnification, and meticulous hemostasis is obtained, with attention to the identification and bipolar cauterization of vessels before their division. As taught by Bunnell, and emphasized by Brand and Hollister,[3] "Every time we clamp or burn a bleeding point, we destroy tissue and leave a scar. Thus the meticulous discipline of the hand surgeon requires that bleeding points be picked up at the exact point and lifted clear of other tissues before they are burned or tied, so that the bulk of dead tissue and the probability of hematoma are both minimized."

After the full-thickness flap is raised off the extensor paratenon, any residual adhesions between the tendon and skin are released sharply. A Freer elevator is helpful in releasing adhesions proximal and distal to the incision. I next sharply release along the palmar aspect of the lateral bands from the base of the proximal phalanx to the mid-portion of the middle phalanx. At the level of the PIP joint, this involves division of the transverse retinacular ligament (**Fig. 3**). This structure overlies the collateral ligament and is very thin. Safe division is facilitated by passing an elevator deep to the lateral band, separating the transverse retinacular ligament from the collaterals. Once the radial and ulnar lateral bands have been released, I work alternately on the radial and ulnar aspects of the finger, using an elevator to release adhesions between the extensor tendon and bone (**Fig. 4**). The elevator should pass without restriction from the base of the proximal phalanx up to the origin of the dorsal capsule, or if a dorsal capsulotomy is performed, to the central slip insertion. In the presence of limited DIP flexion, or active DIP extension, the tenolysis is continued over the middle phalanx to the terminal tendon insertion. Care is taken not to disrupt the central slip and terminal tendon insertions, or the triangular ligament.

At this point, passive motion of the affected joints is assessed, and if full passive motion is present, the tourniquet (if used) is deflated and the patient asked actively to flex and extend their finger. If there continues to be limited active excursion of the tendon, the tendon is explored, extending the incision if necessary and remaining adhesions released. Occasionally, following an adequate tenolysis, manual traction on the tendon produces full extension, but there remains a residual extensor lag when the patient actively extends their finger. This is caused by lengthening of the extensor mechanism from stretch, gap and pseudotendon formation, or apex palmar fracture malunion.[15]

Dorsal Capsulectomy

If there is persistent limitation in passive flexion, a dorsal capsulotomy is required. Often, the dorsal capsule is released from the neck of the proximal phalanx in the process of tenolysing the deep surface of the extensor tendon to the insertion of the central slip. If the dorsal capsule is still intact, it is approached by dorsally retracting the lateral band at the level of the collateral ligament. The radial and ulnar sides of the joint are approached separately, and the dorsal capsule incised transversely from the dorsal margin of the collateral ligament to the midline. A small elevator is now used to release any intra-articular adhesions, and then swept palmarly to mobilize the volar plate and free the retrocondylar fossa. Infrequently, in the setting of persistent limited passive flexion, release of the dorsal fibers of the proper collateral ligament is necessary (**Fig. 5**).

Postoperative Care

Patients start a supervised therapy program the day following extensor tenolysis and dorsal capsulectomy. They are instructed to begin pain medications before their anesthetic wears off, and to maintain a scheduled dosing regimen. Strict elevation is required to minimize edema, which impairs motion, increases pain, and promotes new adhesions. Patients are encouraged to perform active and passive motion exercises on an hourly basis.

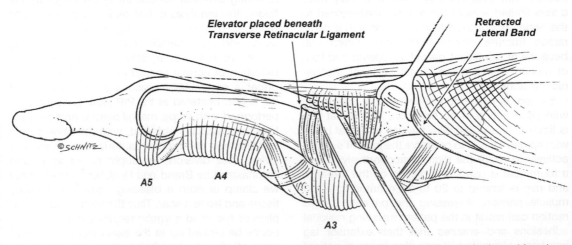

Fig. 3. The deep surface of the extensor mechanism is approached by incising just volar to the lateral bands on the radial and ulnar aspect. At the level of the PIP joint, the transverse retinacular ligament is incised. (*Courtesy of* Gary Schnitz, GSchnitz@ihtsc.com.)

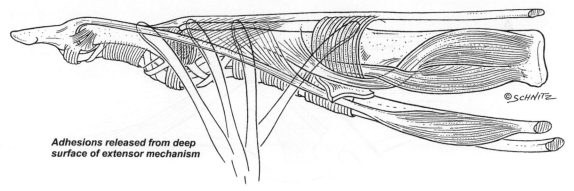

Adhesions released from deep surface of extensor mechanism

Fig. 4. Adhesions to the deep surface of the extensor mechanism are released with an elevator. Care is taken to protect the central slip and terminal tendon insertions. (*Courtesy of* Gary Schnitz, GSchnitz@ihtsc.com.)

In my experience, the extremely motivated patient does their hourly exercises nearly around the clock for the first week or two, and these patients often have the best results. Between exercises, the digits are kept in a static extension gutter splint. Taping and dynamic splinting are initiated, if needed, to improve passive flexion. Additionally, neuromuscular electrical stimulation may be added to maximize tendon excursion. Formal therapy continues daily for the first 1 to 2 weeks, and then continues 3 days a week. As the patients' swelling resolves, and comfortable active motion is gained, the splint is weaned to nighttime only use, typically at 4 to 6 weeks after surgery. During this phase, care is taken to observe for the development of an extensor lag, which necessitates resumption of full-time extension splinting and avoidance of passive flexion for 3 to 7 days.

FLEXOR PHASE

Once the patient's motion has plateaued, and the soft tissues have reached equilibrium (resolution of edema, induration, and so forth), the finger is fully reassessed. The active and passive motion is measured, and sensibility checked. Ideally, the patient has now achieved a satisfactory amount of passive flexion and active extension. If this is not the case, the cause should be identified if possible. This may include poor patient participation; inadequate amount of structured therapy; or patient predisposition (biologic tendency to hypertrophic scar formation, prolonged induration and edema, and so forth). If the cause cannot be corrected or mitigated, further surgical intervention likely proves futile.

Patients with isolated palmar disease, and those who have successful correction of their dorsal disease through therapy or surgery, have Types 3, 5, 6, or 7 digits. The treatment again depends on defining the offending structures, but unfortunately this cannot always be determined preoperatively. Often it is necessary to prepare the patient for several different scenarios, depending on the intraoperative findings. Type 5 digits have flexion contracture and only need palmar capsuloligamentous release. Type 3 digits, in addition to capsuloligamentous release, also need flexor tendon dysfunction addressed, as do Type 6 digits. Treatment of the flexor tendon system may consist of flexor tenolysis alone, tenolysis with pulley reconstruction, one-stage tendon grafting, or two-stage tendon grafting, with the decision often made based on intraoperative findings. For example, even in patients with active excursion of their flexor tendons preoperatively, there may be significant scarring and fraying of the tendons. Following the tenolysis procedure, these tendons may end up reduced in caliber and strength, which requires a more gentle rehabilitation protocol. When severe damage is found, tenolysis with pulley preservation may be technically impossible, and excision of the tendons, pulleys, and staged tendon grafting required.

Flexor Tenolysis

Flexor tenolysis is performed in a similar fashion as extensor tenolysis. If possible, the procedure is performed with a wrist or metacarpal level local anesthetic, with short-acting or no sedation, and limited use of tourniquet. Incisions are made in a Bruner or midlateral fashion. I find both approaches work well, and do not strictly favor one approach. When, based on original injury and preoperative assessment, I think most adhesions are found at or proximal to the flexor digitorum superficialis insertion, I use a Bruner approach. This allows the surgeon to start with a targeted area (eg, A1–A3 pulleys), then extend as needed. When it is likely that the entire sheath

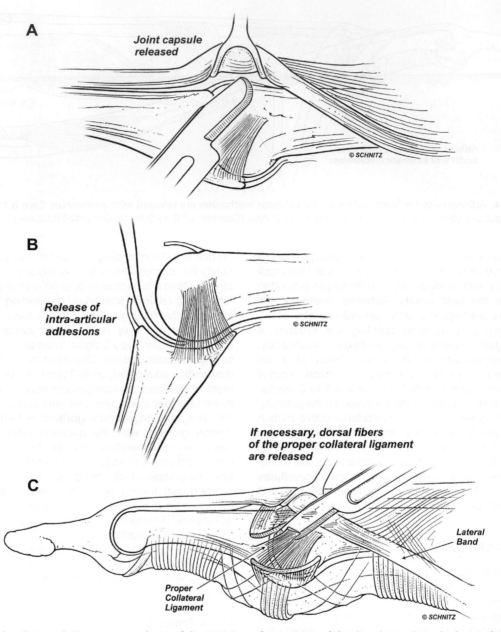

A Joint capsule released

B Release of intra-articular adhesions

C If necessary, dorsal fibers of the proper collateral ligament are released

Lateral Band

Proper Collateral Ligament

Fig. 5. (*A–C*) Capsuloligamentous release of the PIP joint. After incision of the dorsal capsule and release of intra-articular adhesions, the dorsal fibers of the proper collateral ligament may be released, if necessary. (*Courtesy of Gary Schnitz, GSchnitz@ihtsc.com.*)

needs to be exposed, I prefer the midlateral approach, which preserves a healthy skin envelope over the flexor tendons. The main advantage of the midlateral incision is realized in the early postoperative period, an acceptable area for wound dehiscence. Following flexor tenolysis, patients need to begin immediate range of motion exercises for optimal results. The combination of postoperative swelling and early motion can lead to wound dehiscence. In the Brunner incision,

this open wound is often directly over the flexor sheath and tendons, which may necessitate further surgery, whereas in the midlateral approach, the wound opens on the side of the digit, and healing by secondary intention is usually successful.

Again, meticulous soft tissue handling is critical in this demanding procedure. The flexor theca and neurovascular bundles are identified outside the zone of injury, and strict hemostasis obtained as the flaps are elevated. The pulley system is now scrutinized and access to the flexor tendons planned. Ideally the A1, A2, and A4 pulleys are preserved. This is especially true in the small finger, where there is already a relatively narrow A2 pulley, and protection of the A1 pulley maintains optimal function.

I prefer first to expose the flexor tendons just proximal to the A1 pulley and fully release all adhesions at this level. I next establish a window in the flexor sheath from the distal border of the A2 pulley to the proximal border of the A4 pulley (**Fig. 6**). After releasing the extratendonous and intertendonous adhesions at this level, I next free the tendons within the A1 to A2 sheath. This is often the most difficult part of the procedure, because of the decussation of the superficialis. The first step is to release the adhesions between the outer surface of the tendons and the overlying sheath and underlying bone. Specially designed tenolysis knives are commercially available to facilitate this task.[16] Another helpful technique is to pass a suture around the flexor tendons proximal to the A1 pulley (**Fig. 7**). A small hemostat is then passed from the window distal to A2, along the radial aspect of the sheath, to grasp the radial suture limb. The ulnar suture limb is next retrieved, and with alternating tension applied to both limbs, the suture is pulled distally. This acts like a gigili saw to release the adhesions between the tendons and bone, or if the adhesions are strong, the suture delivers the adhesions so that they can be divided under direct visualization.[17]

Finally, intertendonous adhesions between the profundus and superficialis are released. Again, this is facilitated by use of tenolysis knives and suture loops, and differential tension on the tendons. Differential tension is accomplished by placing a longitudinally directed force on the flexors in opposite directions. The profundus is grasped with a moistened sponge or Ragnall retractor proximal to A1, and pulled proximally, while the superficialis is grasped distal to the A2 pulley and pulled distally. The direction of force on each tendon is next switched, pulling the superficialis proximally and the profundus distally. Caution must be taken when pulling on the tendons. If the tendons are pulled too forcefully in a palmar direction, instead of a longitudinal direction, pulley rupture may occur. Excessive longitudinal force is also dangerous, because the tendon can be avulsed from the musculotendonous junction or distal insertion.

At this point, the adequacy of the tenolysis is assessed. Traction on the superficialis proximal to the pulleys should provide flexion of the PIP joint equal to the passive motion. Traction on the profundus should also fully flex the PIP joint and the DIP joint, unless adhesions are present within or distal to the A4 pulley. If present, these adhesions can usually be released from the window created proximal to the A4 pulley. Occasionally, a second window needs to be created from the distal margin of the A4 pulley to the profundus insertion to complete the tenolysis.

The final step is to assess the patient's active motion, if possible. In patients who are unable to generate sufficient active flexion because of tourniquet paresis or those under regional or general anesthesia, a flexor check at the wrist is required. Once the desired tendon is isolated, the wrist is stabilized in extension, and longitudinal traction applied. Full flexion (equal to the passive) should now be present (**Fig. 8**).

Palmar Capsulectomy

Patients with limited passive extension of the PIP joint have capsuloligamentous contracture. The

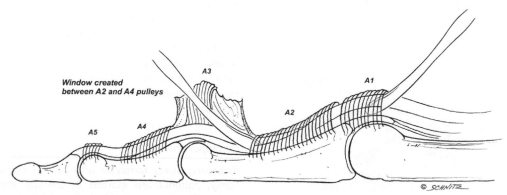

Fig. 6. Approach to flexor tendons. Access to adhesions from the proximal border of the A1 pulley and a window extending from the distal border of the A2 pulley to the proximal border of the A4 pulley. (*Courtesy of* Gary Schnitz, GSchnitz@ihtsc.com.)

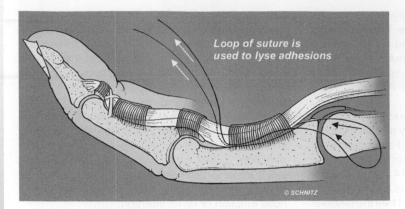

Loop of suture is used to lyse adhesions

© SCHNITZ

Fig. 7. Suture tenolysis. (*Courtesy of Gary Schnitz, GSchnitz@ihtsc. com.*)

structures involved may include the volar plate, checkrein ligaments, accessory collateral, proper collateral ligaments, or arthrofibrosis in isolation or combinations. Patients with limited passive interphalangeal joint extension following flexor tenolysis (Type 1 or Type 3) or patients with isolated flexion contractures (Type 5) are candidates for this procedure.

The procedure can be performed either through a lateral approach, as described by Curtis,[18] or by a palmar approach. Regardless of the skin incision used, the technique of palmar capsulectomy should follow a logical, stepwise sequence. If a flexor tenolysis has been performed, the flexor sheath has already been opened between the A2 and A4 pulleys, in patients without flexor adhesions, creation of a pulley window is the first step, and may alone provide some improvement in joint extension.

The next step is release of the proximal attachments of the volar plate onto the proximal phalanx, the checkrein ligaments. Occasionally, release of

these structures alone allows for full correction of the contracture.[19] The checkrein ligaments are found on the radial and ulnar side of the midline. Each proper digital artery sends a transverse branch, the ladder branch, beneath the checkrein ligament. They meet at the midline and supply the vincula. These should be protected, if possible, and each checkrein ligament is divided distal to the ladder branch. Following release of the proximal attachments of the volar plate, the volar plate is freed from the underlying proximal phalanx, and the joint gently manipulated. If full extension is obtained, the procedure is complete. Frequently, residual contracture persists, and the next step is to release the accessory collateral ligaments at their attachment into the volar plate. The flexor tendons are first retracted to one side of the digit, and the opposite accessory collateral ligament is incised along its' insertion into the volar plate from proximal to the base of the middle phalanx. The tendons are now retracted to the other side of the finger, the opposite accessory collateral released in identical fashion, and the joint gently manipulated into extension.

If there remains a persistent contracture, the last step is release of the proper collateral ligament. This is begun along the volar origin of the ligament, symmetrically, on the radial and ulnar aspects of the finger. The release is continued dorsally, as needed, until full extension is achieved. Full excision of the proper collateral ligament has also been described, and can be performed if necessary.[20]

Postoperative Care

Following flexor tenolysis and palmar capsulectomy, patients are started in therapy immediately. They are educated on strict elevation, maintenance of pain control, and kept in a full extension splint. Therapy begins on the first

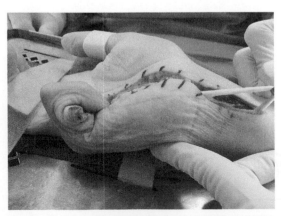

Fig. 8. Traction flexor check at wrist used to assess adequacy of tenolysis in patient unable actively to flex intraoperatively.

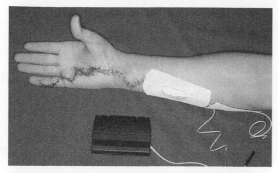

Fig. 9. Use of neuromuscular electric stimulation to maximize excursion of the flexor tendon following tenolysis.

postoperative day and hourly exercises begun. Patients are instructed in both active and passive motion, with an emphasis on full composite flexion and extension; differential tendon gliding; and blocking of the superficialis and profundus tendons (except in the small finger because of risk of rupture). Full passive motion must be regained quickly and then maintained throughout the period of scar maturation and remodeling. Composite taping or dynamic splinting are added to improve passive flexion as necessary, and in patients who are not able to achieve full active pull-through, neuromuscular electrical stimulation is used to obtain supramaximal contraction (**Fig. 9**). Care must be taken, however, in those patients whose flexor tendon quality is poor following tenolysis. These "frayed" tendons must be handled less aggressively, for fear of rupture.[16] As with extensor tenolysis, formal therapy continues daily for the first 1 to 2 weeks, and then continues 3 days a week. The extension splint is weaned beginning at 4 weeks postoperative, and progressive strengthening begun at week 6.

I find it important to review the natural history of scar remodeling with the patient during the postoperative period. I reinforce with them that even after they obtain the motion achieved at surgery, they are at risk of losing it again during the period of scar maturation if they do not continue to maintain their gains on a daily basis. Even 4 to 6 months after surgery, patients frequently find that their fingers are stiff when they wake up, and they need to take 10 to 15 minutes to stretch them out again.

SUMMARY

The stiff finger is a challenging entity for both patient and surgeon. Even with early diagnosis and perfect patient compliance, persistent edema and aggressive scar can still preclude restoration of normal motion. Many stiff fingers are avoidable with appropriate precautions, however, and many of those that become stiff can be improved with aggressive splinting and surgical management. Every hand with an injury should be treated as an injured hand, understanding that the sequelae of even an isolated finger injury often impact the rest of the hand. Immobilization should only be used when necessary, and only for the joints required. Patients need to be educated on what needs to be protected, what is safe to move, and the importance of moving what is allowed, even if it hurts.

Once a contracture is established, aggressive therapy and splinting is often effective in reducing or eliminating the stiffness. Surgery is reserved for recalcitrant contractures in compliant, motivated patients. Preoperative evaluation should determine active and passive motion of involved joints, and all dorsal and palmar pathologies contributing to the stiffness. Classification of the type of motion loss, and knowledge of the dysfunctional structures, then allows one to determine the correct procedure, or sequence of procedures, necessary to restore the finger to optimal function.

REFERENCES

1. Singer AJ, Clark RA. Cutaneous wound healing. N Engl J Med 1999;341(10):738–46.
2. Watson HK, Weinzweig J. Stiff Joints. Green's operative hand surgery. 4th edition. New York: Churchill Livingstone; 1999. p. 552–62.
3. Brand PW, Hollister A. Clinical mechanics of the hand. 3rd edition. St. Louis (MO): Mosby Year Book; 1999.
4. Reish RG, Eriksson E. Scars: a review of emerging and currently available therapies. Plast Reconstr Surg 2008;122(4):1068–78.
5. Meals RA. Posttraumatic limb swelling and joint stiffness are not causally related experimental observations in rabbits. Clin Orthop Relat Res 1993;287: 292–303.
6. Jupiter JB, Goldfarb CA, Nagy L, et al. Posttraumatic reconstruction in the hand. J Bone Joint Surg Am 2007;89(2):428–35.
7. Fetrow KO. Tenolysis in the hand and wrist. A clinical evaluation of two hundred and twenty flexor and extensor tenolyses. J Bone Joint Surg Am 1967; 49(4):667–85.
8. Schneider LH. Flexor tendons: late reconstruction. In: Green DP, Pederson WC, editors. 3rd edition, In: Operative hand surgery, vol. 2. New York: Churchill Livingstone; 1993. p. 1898–949.

9. Fessm EE, Philips CA. Hand splinting: principles and methods. 2nd edition. St. Louis (MO): C.V. Mosby Company; 1987.

10. Prosser R. Splinting in the management of proximal interphalangeal joint flexion contracture. J Hand Ther 1996;9(4):378–86.

11. Scheker LR, Chesher SP, Netscher DT, et al. Functional results of dynamic splinting after transmetacarpal, wrist, and distal forearm replantation. J Hand Surg Br 1995;20(5):584–90.

12. Bonutti PM, Windau JE, Ables BA, et al. Static progressive stretch to reestablish elbow range of motion. Clin Orthop Relat Res 1994;303:128–34.

13. Duncan RM. Basic principles of splinting the hand. Phys Ther 1989;69(12):1104–16.

14. Lalonde D, Bell M, Benoit P, et al. A multicenter prospective study of 3,110 consecutive cases of elective epinephrine use in the fingers and hand: the Dalhousie project clinical phase. J Hand Surg Am 2005;30(5):1061–7.

15. Vahey JW, Wegner DA, Hastings H III. Effect of proximal phalangeal fracture deformity on extensor tendon function. J Hand Surg Am 1998;23(4):673–81.

16. Azari KK, Meals RA. Flexor tenolysis. Hand Clin 2005;21(2):211–7.

17. Idler RS. Flexor tenolysis. Operat Tech Orthop 1998; 8(2):120–6.

18. Curtis RM. Capsulectomy of the interphalangeal joints of the fingers. J Bone Joint Surg Am 1954; 36(6):1219–32.

19. Watson HK, Light TR, Johnson TR. Checkrein resection for flexion contracture of the middle joint. J Hand Surg Am 1979;4(1):67–71.

20. Diao E, Richard GE. Total collateral ligament excision for contractures of the proximal interphalangeal joint. J Hand Surg Am 1993;18(3):395–402.

Complications of Small Joint Arthroplasty

Matthew L. Drake, MD[a,b], Keith A. Segalman, MD[a,c],*

KEYWORDS

- Complications • Fractures • Implant • Pyrocarbon
- Silicone • Small joint arthroplasty

Arthritis in the small joints of the hand can be treated with arthrodesis or arthroplasty. Arthrodesis has known risks of infection, pain, and nonunion. Unfortunately, hand function is severely limited by arthrodesis, particularly in certain joints like the metacarpophalangeal (MCP) joint and the proximal interphalangeal (PIP) joints of the ulnar digits. Arthroplasty has been successful in preserving motion and alleviating pain for the distal interphalangeal (DIP), PIP, and MCP joints. Unfortunately, complications arise that limit the success of surgery. Silicone implants have been reliable for many years but still present with the risks of infection, implant breakage, stiffness, and pain. Newer implant designs may limit some of these complications, but present with unique problems such as dislocations and loosening. The literature is not clear as to which type of implant provides the most reliable results. It is clear that no implant arthroplasty is indicated in the face of active bony infection, poor soft tissue coverage, or a boutonnière or swan-neck deformity.[1,2]

PROXIMAL INTERPHALANGEAL JOINT
Silicone

Silicone implants have been used for the PIP joint for more than 30 years. There are very large series reporting excellent results.[3] In general, very few series report improvement in range of motion after surgery. Pain relief is generally excellent and improvement in function is clear. It is difficult with a radiolucent implant to determine if there is a fracture of the implant. Indirect radiographic parameters include subluxation/dislocation of the joint, subsidence, or bony fracture (**Fig. 1**).

Malalignment after silicone arthroplasty is not a major functional problem unless there is implant fracture. Hage and colleagues[4] reported on 16 implants placed for posttraumatic arthritis with a 4-year follow-up. There was noted to be only a 4° average lateral deviation and 8° of rotational abnormality. Iselin and Conti[5] reported that 2 out of 25 implants with up to 25-year follow-up had deviation of 10° and 15°, respectively. Lin and colleagues' series[6] of 69 implants, inserted for both posttraumatic and inflammatory arthritis, demonstrated no instability and only a 4° average deformity. The investigators emphasized that no collateral reconstruction was necessary. Finally, Adamson and colleagues,[2] in a series of 40 joints, placed only for inflammatory arthritis, reported only 4 of 40 implants with postoperative ulnar drift. One patient did have 30° of ulnar deviation.

The incidence of fracture of the implant is difficult to ascertain but ranges from 5% to 30%. Takigawa and colleagues[1] reported the results on 70 implants followed for an average of 6.5 years. These investigators reported 11 of 70 clear fractures and 16 of 70 suspected fractures for an

The authors did not receive any outside funding or grants in support of this work.

a The Curtis National Hand Center, Union Memorial Hospital, 3333 North Calvert Street, #200, Baltimore, MD 21218, USA
b Walter Reed Army Medical Center, 6900 Georgia Avenue NW, Washington, DC 20307, USA
c The Johns Hopkins School of Medicine, Baltimore, MD 21287, USA
* Corresponding author. The Curtis National Hand Center, Union Memorial Hospital, 3333 North Calvert Street, #200, Baltimore, MD 21218.
E-mail address: ksegalman@comcast.net

Hand Clin 26 (2010) 205–212
doi:10.1016/j.hcl.2010.01.003

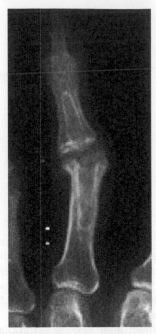

Fig. 1. Presumed fracture of a PIP silicone implant based on subluxation and deformity of the joint.

overall incidence of 30%. Ashworth and colleagues[7] noted only a 10% incidence of fracture in 99 implants looked at nearly 6 years after insertion for rheumatoid arthritis. Iselin and Conti[5] noted 5 fractures in 25 implants followed for up to 25 years. Lin and colleagues[6] noted only 5 fractures out of 69 implants followed for an average of 3.4 years.

Even when a fracture does not occur after implant insertion, there are radiographic changes that are worrisome (**Fig. 2**). Adamson and colleagues' review[2] of 40 joints demonstrated sclerotic lines around the implant in 17 digits (43%), each associated with a 25° loss of motion. Ashworth and colleagues[7] found in a series of 99 implants that 78% had sclerosis and 12% had bony resorption at 2 years. Silicone synovitis is extremely rare. Throughout the literature only Takigawa and colleagues[1] mention 3 cases of silicone synovitis.

A few series address the effect of surgical approach on complication rate. Lin and colleagues' series[6] included only those implants placed through an anterior approach, the series by Adamson and colleagues[2] and Namdari and Weiss[8] included only a dorsal approach, and Takigawa and colleagues[1] reviewed implants through a variety of approaches. It is not possible to see any comparative differences between these publications. Horton and Dimmen[9] directly compared the results between a dorsal and volar insertion in

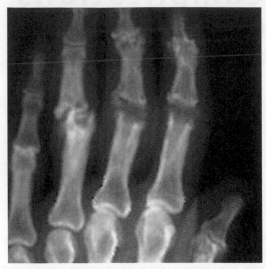

Fig. 2. Sclerosis around PIP silicone implant.

59 implants reviewed up to 5 years after insertion. Four of 21 patients required revision because of excess bone buildup in the dorsal approach, but no difference was found in implant fracture. This result is not conclusive proof as to which approach has the least complications, although the volar approach seems to have fewer complications. Excellent range of motion has been reported with a lateral approach, but there are no comparative series with the other approaches (**Fig. 3**).[10]

Pyrocarbon

There has been recent interest in pyrocarbon implants. The pyrocarbon implant demonstrates a modulus of elasticity similar to that of cortical bone, which may allow for better stress transfer at the bone-implant interface (**Fig. 4**A and B).[11] Unfortunately, the implant requires adequate soft tissue support to prevent subluxation or dislocation, as well as preoperative alignment (**Fig. 5**). There is one report of a stem fracture during insertion.[12] The implant is not indicated if collateral

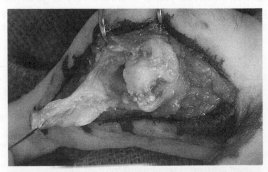

Fig. 3. Lateral approach for insertion of a PIP silicone implant.

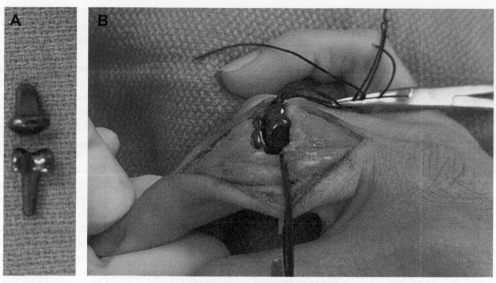

Fig. 4. Pyrocarbon implant. (*A*) The implant. (*B*) The implant placed in situ.

ligament support is not present. The manufacturers initially stated that the implant had the potential for bony ingrowth, but recent studies have confirmed that no bony ingrowth occurs between pyrocarbon and the surrounding bone.[13] Bravo and colleagues, Nunley and colleagues, and Tuttle and Stern[13–15] have reported on retrospective series of patients who have pyrocarbon implants inserted for PIP arthritis.

Bravo and colleagues[14] presented the first large series of pyrocarbon implants. These investigators presented 50 implants inserted through a dorsal central slip splitting approach. The average postoperative range of motion was 47°. There was a 79% satisfaction rate, but 40% of the implants shifted; 28% had additional surgery for instability, loosening, stiffness, deformity, or pain. Eight percent of the patients had revision arthroplasty, and 2 patients even elected to have an amputation.

Tuttle and Stern[13] presented another more recent retrospective series of patients with pyrocarbon implants. Eighteen patients were evaluated an average of 13 months after insertion. All implants were inserted through a dorsal approach using a "Chamay" approach of preserving the central slip insertion. There was no change in the total arc of motion, but the movement was shifted into a more flexed posture. Four implants were inserted with an angulatory deformity averaging 12°, and all implants had radiolucent lines around the implant without gross loosening. Only 7 of 18 were free from pain, contracture, loosening, and deformity at follow-up. Squeaking in the joint was reported in 8 of 18 patients. Postinsertion squeaking has no definitive explanation; however, excessive soft tissue tightness across the joint may be a contributing factor. Squeaking has been postulated to contribute to aseptic loosening of the implant (**Fig. 6**).

Dislocations have been reported by Tuttle and Stern[13] and Chung and colleagues.[16] These investigators treated the dislocation successfully with closed reduction and immobilization. Revision surgery has also been performed required secondary to persistent instability. Joint contracture is another well-described problem after pyrocarbon implant arthroplasty. Tuttle and Stern[13] described 5 of 18 patients with less than 35° of motion, and Nunley and colleagues[15] described 1 in 7 patients with a fixed boutonnière deformity after multiple revisions. Contracture may occur less frequently using a volar approach to insert the implant, thereby avoiding damage to the central slip. The manufacturer provides a specialized jig for making the oblique cut in the proximal phalanx through a volar approach.

In light of numerous complications, it is easy to question whether there is a role for the pyrocarbon

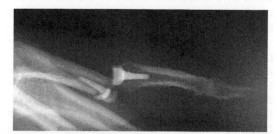

Fig. 5. Dorsal dislocation of a pyrocarbon PIP implant.

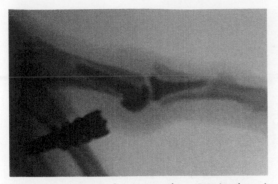

Fig. 6. Loosening of a pyrocarbon PIP implant in a patient with a long history of "squeaking."

implant. Branam and colleagues[17] reported a retrospective review of silicone and pyrocarbon implants. Twenty silicone and 19 pyrocarbon implants were followed for an average of 45 and 19 months, respectively. Angulatory deformity was present in 16 of 22 silicone implants and in 5 of 19 pyrocarbon implants. The minor complication rate was 14% for silicone implants versus 32% for pyrocarbon implants, but the major complication rate was 22% for silicone implants and 0% for the pyrocarbon implants. Subsidence was much higher in the silicone implant than the pyrocarbon implants, and 8 of the 18 pyrocarbon implants squeaked.

The senior author's own series comparing silicone and pyrocarbon implants showed slightly different results. A retrospective review of 20 silicone and 15 pyrocarbon implants implanted mostly for osteoarthritis and posttraumatic arthritis found an equal complication rate of 32% in both groups. Additional surgery was required in 14% of the joints in both groups. The main difference is the time for revision: 71 months after silicone insertion and 11 months for a pyrocarbon implant (Segalman, unpublished data, 2007).

Squitieri and Chung[18] also reported a high revision rate of 33% as compared with the 13% revision rate reported by Wijk and colleagues[19] with the use of pyrocarbon PIP implants. Despite the high revision rate with pyrocarbon PIP implants, these investigators believe that the implant has a certain defined role. The pyrocarbon implant is best for a young patient with posttraumatic arthritis with no angulatory deformity and adequate soft tissue coverage.

Other Implants

A variety of other metal and plastic implants have been developed for use in the PIP joints. Linscheid and colleagues[20] published a 14-year experience with cemented surface replacement arthroplasty. Out of 66 implanted prostheses, there were 5

cases of instability, 5 swan-neck deformities, 1 intraoperative fracture, 12 reoperations, and 7 cases of malalignment. Although the investigators do not report a major complication rate, it certainly seems higher than the reported results with other prostheses. Osteointegrated prostheses have been reported by Moller and colleagues and Lundborg and Branemark.[21–23] In an initial series of 22 implants, 4 of 22 fractured, 27% deformed, and 2 required revision.[21] A later series from 2004 reported 94% had complete osteointegration of the prosthesis, but nearly a quarter of the patients had loosening.[22] Lundborg and Branemark[23] followed 25 osteointegrated implants with an 8.5-year follow-up. Although 94% of the implants integrated into bone, 68% of the spacers fractured and 11 joints had to be revised. It appears from other studies that cementing makes a difference in bony fixation but not in the complication rate.

Comparing the loosening rate of cemented and uncemented prostheses, Jennings and Livingstone[24] found a loosening rate of 4% in cemented prostheses and 39% of uncemented prostheses. Johnstone and colleagues[25] also found a higher complication rate in the uncemented group. In a review of 27 CoCr and ultrahigh molecular weight polyethylene (UHMWPE) implants, there were 2 of 27 (8%) failures in the cemented group and 5 of 21 (26%) failures in the uncemented group. Sauerbier and colleagues[26] did not separate cemented and noncemented UHMWPE and titanium implants, but 8 out of 82 implants had instability and 12 out of 82 implants required secondary procedures. The indications for using metal and plastic PIP implants are not clear, but clearly uncemented implants have a higher complication rate.

Ceramic prostheses have been reported by Pettersson and colleagues and Hobby and colleagues.[27,28] Pettersson and colleagues[28] reported on a group of 20 implants with only 1-year follow-up. No patients required revision surgery, but 2 of 20 implants were clearly loose. Hobby and colleagues[27] reported on a much larger group of patients, 164 implants, with much longer follow-up (up to 5 years' follow-up). There was unfortunately a 29% revision rate and an additional 20% failure rate. Based on the limited data, these investigators cannot recommend ceramic implants.

Despite the high complication rates, PIP arthroplasty is clearly indicated for painful joints associated with limited motion and failure of conservative treatment. Silicone is the most reliable for deformed joints, that is, those with any subluxation, especially in older patients. Pyrocarbon is best for the stable joint in a younger patient, and the authors cannot recommend ceramic or integrated prostheses until more research is completed.

METACARPOPHALANGEAL JOINT

Implant arthroplasty has also been extensively reported for treating painful MCP joints. Several varieties of implants have been used ranging from traditional silicone, to a modified silicone prosthesis, to pyrocarbon implants.

Silicone

The earliest report including complication data regarding silicone implants was published by Swanson and colleagues in 1986.[3] This radiographic study examined the findings in 133 joints followed over 5 years. The investigators found that bony changes around the implants were exceedingly common. It was observed that the distal metacarpal metaphyseal cortical thickness increased an average of 114% and the proximal phalanx metaphyseal cortical thickness increased by 85%. In addition, an average loss of 9% of metacarpal length was observed. No comment was made as to whether these findings had any clinical significance. Ten implants were found to have fractured for a rate of 7%. The need for revision was not specified in this report.

Goldfarb and Stern[29] reported on the long-term outcomes of silicone arthroplasty in rheumatoid patients in 2003. This case series followed 208 MCP joint arthroplasties in 36 patients with 14-year follow-up. These investigators found an implant fracture rate of 63%, with an additional 22% of implants severely deformed at final follow-up. It was also noted that 29% of the joints had developed peri-implant bony erosions, with the majority of metacarpals and proximal phalanges showing a moderate loss of length.

Instability after silicone implants has been a major concern, particularly in the rheumatoid population. Results traditionally have been worse in the ulnar digits for instability and range of motion. However, in a recent prospective multicenter study, Chung and colleagues[30] demonstrated that digits up to 1 year after silicone implant arthroplasty for rheumatoid arthritis do better in the ulnar digits than radially. In addition, the greatest improvement in range of motion was ulnar, not radially.

More recently, investigators have reported on a new variety of silicone implant with an anatomically shaped contour of 30° of flexion built into the prosthesis. In 2009, Namdari and Weiss[8] reported on the Neuflex silicone implant for osteoarthritis of the MCP joint in 13 joints with 4-year follow-up. An extension lag at the PIP joint was found in 6 of the 13 digits. Only 1 implant fracture was noted at 58 months. Ulnar deviation was minimal in most patients, with a range of 0° to 15°. Only 1 patient underwent revision at 7 years at the time of an adjacent digit arthroplasty.

Kimani and colleagues[31] reported a much larger series of Neuflex implants in 2009, comprising the outcomes for 237 implants in 66 patients with 7-year follow-up. These investigators found a survivorship of 88%, although there was a 32% rate of implant fracture. Sixteen implants required revision: 7 for deformity, 7 for fracture, 1 for dislocation, and 1 for bony impingement.

Two studies have reported comparing traditional silicone prostheses with the Neuflex implant. Delaney and colleagues[32] first reported a double-blind trial comparing these implants in 2005. Thirty-seven Swanson implants were compared with 40 Neuflex implants with 2-year follow-up. Unfortunately, no complication data were reported. Pettersson and colleagues[28] reported data comparing these 2 implants in 2006. This study included 40 patients with 156 joints randomized to the 2 implants with 1-year follow-up. The investigators found a fracture rate of 6% in the traditional silicone group versus 2% in the Neuflex group, although statistical significance was not noted. Two of the Neuflex group subluxated and 2 patients with Sutter implants demonstrated massive heterotopic ossification. No reoperations were performed at final follow-up.

Most surgeons do not think of using silicone implants for the thumb MCP joint in rheumatoid arthritis, but Figgie and colleagues[33] reported surprisingly good results. After 6.5 years, 42 of 43 joints remained intact with only 1 implant requiring revision for instability. The investigators experienced 1 superficial wound infection and found no evidence of any implant fractures. Their radiographic analysis found a 12% rate of bony resorption around the implants and a 64% rate of peri-implant sclerosis. The clinical significance of this finding was not noted.

Pyrocarbon

Metacarpophalangeal joint arthroplasty has also been attempted with the use of pyrocarbon implants. The use of a noncemented hemispherical pyrocarbon implant was reported by Cook and colleagues[34] in a long-term follow-up case series in 1999. This report included 151 implants in 53 patients over an 8-year period. Thirty-four percent of their patients died before final follow-up, but the implants had been in place for over 7 years prior to death. Eighteen implants in 11 patients required revision for an overall complication rate of 12%. The most common reasons for revision were subluxation, stiffness, and dislocation. One implant was revised for fracture. The investigators did not observe any instances of reactive synovitis. Radiographic analysis revealed a common finding of sclerosis around the implants, and 64% of implants had some degree of subsidence. Survivorship analysis revealed an annual failure rate of 2.1%, with a 16-year survivorship of 70.3%.

In 2007, Parker and colleagues[35] reviewed the early results of a newer design of unconstrained pyrocarbon MCP joint implant. The newer design featured changes to the stem and joint surface contour, as well as structural changes to the material itself. Of these implants, 142 were placed in 61 patients with 1-year follow-up. Of the patients with osteoarthritis, there were 2 minor complications and 2 major complications (extensor tendon rupture and chronic pain requiring implant removal). In the rheumatoid group there were 2 minor complications and 8 major complications (2 subluxations, 1 dislocation requiring revision, severe stiffness, and periprosthetic fracture). In the nonrheumatoid arthritis/osteoarthritis group there were 3 complications (intraoperative fracture, subluxations). The overall complication rate was 14%.

The indications for a pyrocarbon implant are not clear, but the authors do not believe that it is wise to use the implant in the face of inflammatory arthritis. There are no side-by-side comparisons between pyrocarbon and silicone implants.

Alternative Prostheses

Derkash and colleagues[36] reported the outcomes of a combined silicone-Dacron MCP joint implant in 1986. This study included 89 joints in 16 patients with an 11.5-year follow-up. Instability was a major problem with this particular implant. Of the joints, 43% demonstrated greater than 75% palmar subluxation radiographically while 58% of the joints had clinical palmar instability. Ulnar drift proved to be problematic as well, with 36% of the implants having more than 20° of drift. In addition, radiographically 87% of the joints demonstrated some degree of bony destruction. The investigators reported an overall complication rate of 12%, with 4 implants requiring revision for instability, implant fracture in 4 cases, bony destruction in 1 case, and prosthesis "buckling" in 1 case.

Lundborg and colleagues[37] reported on the outcomes of another variety of silicone prosthesis in 1993. This prosthesis had the traditional silicone spacer with metallic osteointegrated intramedullary screws proximally and distally. Their study included 68 joints in 31 patients with 2.5-year follow-up. The investigators did not find any evidence of screw loosening, although a small area of bone resorption around the spacer was generally seen; they noted 4 spacer fractures for an overall fracture rate of 6%.

A less commonly used implant was reported on by Devas and Shah in 1975.[38] This study described the results of a cemented Link Arthroplasty for the MCP joint in 28 patients with 54 joints at 18-month follow-up. Devas and Shah reported 2 infections and 2 implants lost to "necrosing arteritis" in one patient with severe rheumatoid arthritis. One implant dislocated and was managed successfully with closed reduction. One implant fractured at final follow-up.

Other Implants

An uncemented surfaced replacement was reported by Harris and Dias in 2003.[39] This prosthesis was used in 13 joints in 8 patients with a 5-year follow-up. One patient experienced a deep infection necessitating the removal of 2 implants. One implant settled 2 mm radiographically with unknown clinical significance. One implant was malpositioned on the metacarpal side in extension, although no functional problem resulted.

Overall, many varieties of MCP joint arthroplasty have been reported. Complications have been experienced with all prostheses, and none have been shown to be superior in this regard. Despite many varieties of implants used for the MCP joint, silicone seems to be the most reliable, with the fewest complications.

DISTAL INTERPHALANGEAL JOINT

Arthroplasty of the DIP joint is a much less commonly reported procedure. A review of the literature reveals very few case series describing this operation. Of the series available, the investigators describe using a flexible silicone joint implant placed through a dorsal approach. This technique requires incising and repair of extensor tendon. Snow and colleagues[40] published a series of 7 joints replaced in 4 hands in 1977 for osteoarthritis. These investigators advocated the procedure; however, no length of follow-up was given and there were no remarks on complications.

Wilgis[41] reported the largest series of DIP joint arthroplasty in 1997. Eighteen patients received 31 silicone implants, with a 90% survivorship rate reported at 10 years. The most common complication was lateral instability in 52% of the joints; however, Wilgis reported that this was not clinically significant in most patients. One patient developed a recurrent paronychia with concomitant extensor lag. Three implants were removed: 1 due to implant erosion through the dorsal skin, 1 for infection, and 1 for fracture of the implant.

Brown[42] observed similar results in an additional case series published in 1989. In this series, 21 joints underwent silicone arthroplasty in 12 patients. At 26-month follow-up only 1 implant had been removed, because of erosion through the distal phalanx leading to deep infection. This case was salvaged by eventual arthrodesis. Of note, Brown reported that no implant fractures or reactive synovitis were seen.

With so little literature, it is difficult to make strong recommendations. Implant arthroplasty to the DIP joint appears to be indicated in patients with osteoarthritis, pain, limited motion, and those not willing to accept an arthrodesis, although its superiority to arthrodesis is unproven.

SUMMARY

All implants in each joint can lead to complications. Although not proven in the literature, implant arthroplasty does give better function than arthrodesis. Despite the risks of implant fracture and instability, silicone arthroplasty does not lead to silicone synovitis and is a reliable procedure. Pyrocarbon implants are showing some promise, particularly in the osteoarthritic patient. It is too early to make predictions regarding the use of other implants until more long-term studies are published.

REFERENCES

1. Takigawa S, Meletiou S, Sauerbier M, et al. Long-term assessment of Swanson implant arthroplasty in the proximal interphalangeal joint of the hand. J Hand Surg 2004;29A:785–95.
2. Adamson GJ, Gellman H, Brumfield RH Jr, et al. Flexible implant resection arthroplasty of the proximal interphalangeal joint in patients with systemic inflammatory arthritis. J Hand Surg Am 1994;19: 378–84.
3. Swanson AB, Poitevin LA, de Groot SG, et al. Bone remodeling phenomena in flexible implant arthroplasty in the metacarpophalangeal joints. Long-term study. Clin Orthop Relat Res 1986;205: 254–67.
4. Hage JJ, Yoe EP, Zevering JP, et al. Proximal interphalangeal joint silicone arthroplasty for posttraumatic arthritis. J Hand Surg 1999;24A: 73–7.
5. Iselin F, Conti E. Long-term results of proximal interphalangeal joint resection arthroplasties with a silicone implant. J Hand Surg Am 1995;20:S95–7.
6. Lin HH, Wyrick JD, Stern PJ. Proximal interphalangeal joint silicone replacement arthroplasty: clinical results using an anterior approach. J Hand Surg 1995;20A:123–32.
7. Ashworth CR, Hansraj KK, Todd AO, et al. Swanson proximal interphalangeal joint arthroplasty in patients with rheumatoid arthritis. Clin Orthop Relat Res 1997;342:34–7.
8. Namdari S, Weiss AP. Anatomically neutral silicone small joint arthroplasty for osteoarthritis. J Hand Surg Am 2009;34:292–300.
9. Herren DB, Simmen BR. Palmar approach in flexible implant arthroplasty of the proximal interphalangeal joint. Clin Orthop Relat Res 2000; 371:131–5.
10. Segalman KA. Lateral approach to proximal interphalangeal joint implant arthroplasty. J Hand Surg 2007;32A:905–8.
11. Cook SD, Klawitter JJ, Weinstein AM. The influence of implant elastic modulus on the stress distribution around LTI carbon and aluminum oxide dental implants. J Biomed Mater Res 1981;15:879–87.
12. Skie M, Gove N, Ciocanel D. Intraoperative fracture of a pyrocarbon PIP total joint-a case report. Hand (NY) 2007;2:90–3.
13. Tuttle HG, Stern PJ. Pyrolytic carbon proximal interphalangeal joint resurfacing arthroplasty. J Hand Surg Am 2006;31:930–9.
14. Bravo CJ, Rizzo M, Hormel KB, et al. Pyrolytic carbon proximal interphalangeal joint arthroplasty: results with minimum two-year follow-up evaluation. J Hand Surg Am 2007;32:1–11.
15. Nunley RM, Boyer MI, Goldfarb CA. Pyrolytic carbon arthroplasty for posttraumatic arthritis of the proximal interphalangeal joint. J Hand Surg Am 2006; 31:1468–74.
16. Chung KC, Ram AN, Shauver MJ. Outcomes of pyrolytic carbon arthroplasty for the proximal interphalangeal joint. Plast Reconstr Surg 2009;123: 1521–32.
17. Branam BR, Tuttle HG, Stern PJ, et al. Resurfacing arthroplasty versus silicone arthroplasty for proximal interphalangeal joint osteoarthritis. J Hand Surg Am 2007;32:775–88.
18. Squitieri L, Chung KC. A systematic review of outcomes and complications of vascularized toe joint transfer, silicone arthroplasty, and pyrocarbon arthroplasty for posttraumatic joint reconstruction of the finger. Plast Reconstr Surg 2008;121: 1697–707.
19. Wijk U, Wollmark M, Kopylov P, et al. Outcomes of proximal interphalangeal joint pyrocarbon implants. J Hand Surg Am 2010;35:38–43.
20. Linscheid RL, Murray PM, Vidal MA, et al. Development of a surface replacement arthroplasty for proximal interphalangeal joints. J Hand Surg Am 1997; 22:286–98.

21. Moller K, Sollerman C, Geijer M, et al. Early results with osseointegrated proximal interphalangeal joint prostheses. J Hand Surg Am 1999;24:267–74.

22. Moller K, Geijer M, Sollerman C, et al. Radiographic evaluation of osseointegration and loosening of titanium implants in the MCP and PIP joints. J Hand Surg Am 2004;29:32–8.

23. Lundborg G, Branemark PI. Osseointegrated proximal interphalangeal joint prostheses with a replaceable flexible joint spacer—long-term results. Scand J Plast Reconstr Surg Hand Surg 2000;34:345–53.

24. Jennings CD, Livingstone DP. Surface replacement arthroplasty of the proximal interphalangeal joint using the PIP-SRA implant: results, complications, and revisions. J Hand Surg Am 2008;33:1565, e1–11.

25. Johnstone BR, Fitzgerald M, Smith KR, et al. Cemented versus uncemented surface replacement arthroplasty of the proximal interphalangeal joint with a mean 5-year follow-up. J Hand Surg Am 2008;33:726–32.

26. Sauerbier M, Cooney WP, Linscheid RL. Operative technique of surface replacement arthroplasty of the proximal interphalangeal joint. Tech Hand Up Extrem Surg 2001;5:141–7.

27. Hobby JL, Edwards S, Field J, et al. A report on the early failure of the LPM proximal interphalangeal joint replacement. J Hand Surg Eur Vol 2008;33:526–7.

28. Pettersson K, Wagnsjo P, Hulin E. NeuFlex compared with Sutter prostheses: a blind, prospective, randomised comparison of Silastic metacarpophalangeal joint prostheses. Scand J Plast Reconstr Surg Hand Surg 2006;40:284–90.

29. Goldfarb CA, Stern PJ. Metacarpophalangeal joint arthroplasty in rheumatoid arthritis. A long-term assessment. J Bone Joint Surg Am 2003;85: 1869–78.

30. Chung KC, Kotsis SV, Wilgis EF, et al. Outcomes of silicone arthroplasty for rheumatoid metacarpophalangeal joints stratified by fingers. J Hand Surg Am 2009;34:1647–52.

31. Kimani BM, Trail IA, Hearnden A, et al. Survivorship of the Neuflex silicone implant in MCP joint replacement. J Hand Surg Eur Vol 2009;34:25–8.

32. Delaney R, Trail IA, Nuttall D. A comparative study of outcome between the Neuflex and Swanson metacarpophalangeal joint replacements. J Hand Surg Br 2005;30:3–7.

33. Figgie MP, Inglis AE, Sobel M, et al. Metacarpalphalangeal joint arthroplasty of the rheumatoid thumb. J Hand Surg Am 1990;15:210–6.

34. Cook SD, Beckenbaugh RD, Redondo J, et al. Long-term follow-up of pyrolytic carbon metacarpophalangeal implants. J Bone Joint Surg Am 1999;81:635–48.

35. Parker WL, Rizzo M, Moran SL, et al. Preliminary results of nonconstrained pyrolytic carbon arthroplasty for metacarpophalangeal joint arthritis. J Hand Surg Am 2007;32:1496–505.

36. Derkash RS, Niebauer JJ Jr, Lane CS. Long-term follow-up of metacarpal phalangeal arthroplasty with silicone Dacron prostheses. J Hand Surg Am 1986;11:553–8.

37. Lundborg G, Branemark PI, Carlsson I. Metacarpophalangeal joint arthroplasty based on the osseointegration concept. J Hand Surg 1993;18B:693–703.

38. Devas M, Shah V. Link arthroplasty of the metacarpophalangeal joints. A preliminary report of a new method. J Bone Joint Surg Br 1975;57:72–7.

39. Harris D, Dias JJ. Five-year results of a new total replacement prosthesis for the finger metacarpophalangeal joints. J Hand Surg Br 2003;28:432–8.

40. Snow JW, Boyes JG Jr, Greider JL Jr. Implant arthroplasty of the distal interphalangeal joint of the finger for osteoarthritis. Plast Reconstr Surg 1977; 60:558–60.

41. Wilgis EF. Distal interphalangeal joint silicone interpositional arthroplasty of the hand. Clin Orthop Relat Res 1997;342:38–41.

42. Brown LG. Distal interphalangeal joint flexible implant arthroplasty. J Hand Surg Am 1989;14: 653–6.

Complications of Wrist Arthroplasty

Brian D. Adams, MD

KEYWORDS

• Wrist arthroplasty • Risks • Management • Complications

RATIONALE

Normal wrist motion is accomplished by a complex interaction of multiple articulations, which cannot be precisely duplicated by a prosthesis. Thus, every past and present implant design includes a variety of compromises in motion, strength, and durability compared with the natural wrist joint. To optimize the goal to achieve a pain-free, stable, and durable wrist replacement requires proper patient selection, careful preoperative planning, and accurate implantation. Because arthroplasty carries the risks of bearing wear and implant loosening, low-demand patients with special needs or desires for wrist motion are the best candidates. In the past, these were typically patients with rheumatoid arthritis with multiple joint involvement. However, many of these patients have poor bone stock and severe deformity that substantially increase the risk of implant loosening and wrist imbalance.[1] Patients with osteoarthritis and posttraumatic arthritis who are willing to permanently restrict their lifestyle may chose arthroplasty over arthrodesis to perform vocational and avocational activities requiring high dexterity but low stress. These patients often have good bone quality and satisfactory wrist alignment. Thus, multiple factors affect the outcome of total wrist arthroplasty; the most important are physical activity demands of the patient, wrist joint alignment, bone quality, and muscle and tendon function.

HISTORICAL PERSPECTIVE

Swanson[2] designed the first wrist implant to be used in clinical practice in the United States. Although initial clinical results were promising, implant subsidence and breakage were common. Breakage rates were as high as 52% at 72 months.[3] Silicone synovitis also became an important issue, although the incidence was lower than with carpal implants.[3,4]

Early articulated total wrist prostheses incorporated bearings with small surface areas to maximize joint motion, however instability and imbalance were serious problems.[3,5] Various stem designs for fixation in the radius and carpus were tried. Carpal components were typically fixed in the metacarpal canals with cement. A high incidence of loosening marked by metacarpal erosion and implant penetration occurred (**Fig. 1**). Periprosthetic bone resorption of the distal radius was also common.[6] Initial design changes focused on reducing wrist imbalance and distal component loosening by more accurately reproducing normal wrist kinematics through changes in the articulation's position and constraint. The revised Meuli, Trispherical, revised Voltz, and Biaxial prostheses each provided satisfactory early clinical results but follow-up revealed continued problems with imbalance, subsidence, and loosening.[6–12] Menon's[13] prosthesis introduced the concept of augmenting distal component fixation using screws into the carpus combined with an intercarpal fusion. The fixation method proved to be much more durable than previous methods but the bearing design was prone to instability (**Fig. 2**).

The overall experience with different designs during the last 35 years strongly indicates there are specific criteria to optimize the clinical results.[14] Distal component fixation should be primarily within the carpus and not rely on the metacarpal canals. Perhaps of most importance is a solid intercarpal fusion to provide broad support for the component. Using screws to

Department of Orthopaedic Surgery, University of Iowa Hospitals and Clinics, 200 Hawkins Drive, 01077 JPP, Iowa City, IA 52242-1088, USA
E-mail address: brian-d-adams@uiowa.edu

Hand Clin 26 (2010) 213–220
doi:10.1016/j.hcl.2010.01.006
0749-0712/10/$ – see front matter © 2010 Elsevier Inc. All rights reserved.

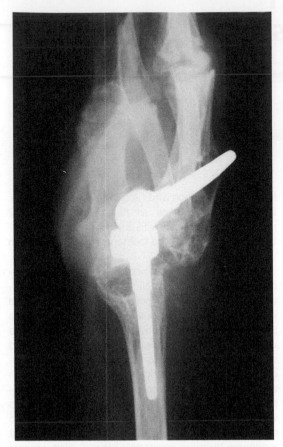

Fig. 1. Biaxial implant with distal component migration resulting in penetration through the dorsal aspect of the third metacarpal.

augment initial fixation has been shown to be effective.[15] The radial component should be shaped to minimize bone resection and preserve the joint capsule to enhance prosthetic stability and wrist balance. Fixation by osteointegration rather than cement would seem to be better for both components to improve durability and reduce bone destruction if revision is necessary. The articulation should be broad, generally ellipsoidal in shape, and semi-constrained to provide a functional range of motion and yet resist imbalance and instability to allow early recovery and durability.[14]

INDICATIONS

The ideal candidate for a total wrist arthroplasty is a patient with a low-demand physical lifestyle who is seeking pain relief and modest wrist motion for ease of function during nonstressful activities. Patients with rheumatoid or osteoarthritis are typical candidates, however the cause of arthritis is much less important than the future stresses

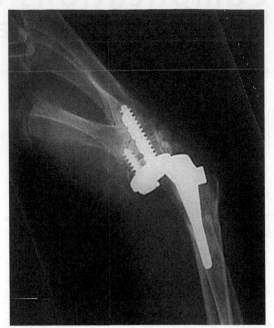

Fig. 2. Universal implant shown with volar dislocation.

the wrist will bear and the quality of the bone and soft tissues before surgery.

In patient selection, it is perhaps more important to consider contraindications rather than indications. Many patients with posttraumatic arthritis are young and active and not candidates for arthroplasty because of the high stresses imposed on the wrist. Likewise, patients with osteoarthritis who have been active in physically demanding activities for many years may not be willing to alter their lifestyle. Patients with rheumatoid arthritis with highly active synovitis that is producing severe bony erosions or joint hyperlaxity have a high risk for implant loosening and are better treated by arthrodesis. Regular use of the upper extremities for support during ambulation or transfers is a contraindication, however intermittent use of crutches or a cane may be acceptable if the patient uses a wrist splint.

Lower extremity surgery such as total hip or knee arthroplasty should be done before wrist replacement to avoid weight bearing on the wrist replacement during rehabilitation. Procedures on the digits should be completed after wrist arthroplasty to optimize joint alignment and tendon tension in the hand.

There must be adequate bone stock and quality to support the implant, especially the carpal component. Implantation in patients with severe osteopenia, bone erosion, or joint deformity is more challenging and the implant fixation is much less durable. Previous surgical fusion or proximal row carpectomy are relative contraindications; these patients must have adequate carpus remaining and intact wrist extensors to convert to an arthroplasty.

POTENTIAL COMPLICATIONS

Potential intraoperative complications include fractures and tendon injury. Early postoperative complications include wound-healing problems (hematoma, wound edge necrosis, dehiscence), extensor tendon adhesions, wrist stiffness, wrist imbalance, distal radioulnar joint problems (impingement, instability, arthrosis), prosthetic instability, and infection. The most common long-term complication is implant loosening, particularly of the distal component in the newer designs. Each of these complications is described along with techniques to minimize the risks and treat the complications.

Intraoperative Fracture

Fluoroscopy is helpful to ensure accurate bone preparation and prosthetic implantation. Preparation of the radius for component implantation requires identification of the central intramedullary canal of the radius and broaching to a press fit for the final component. If the cortical bone is weakened from synovitis or the canal is not fully prepared, implantation of the radial component can cause fracture. To avoid fracture, it is imperative to properly align the radial broaches in the medullary canal and to fully seat trial components with minimal force. If a radius fracture occurs, circumferential cerclage wire(s) can be used to reapproximate and reinforce the shaft and metaphysis. Additional bone graft is placed within the radius canal if needed. A much less stressful rehabilitation program should be pursued to allow bone healing, however the final range of motion is likely to be reduced because of capsular stiffness or tendon adhesions. If initial solid fixation cannot be achieved on the operating table then cement fixation should be used, which also allows for more rapid rehabilitation.

The carpal component is typically fixed by a short stem and screws, which requires precise drilling for proper implant alignment and bone contact. If a carpal fracture occurs, the defect is augmented with bone grafting and longer screws are used that span the fractured area. If the screws extend into a base of the metacarpal on the ulnar side of the wrist, the carpometacarpal (CMC) joint should be prepared for fusion by removing the joint cartilage and inserting cancellous bone graft.

Cement is considered for stem fixation if bone contact around the stem is inadequate or the bone is osteopenic.

Intraoperative Tendon Lacerations

Tendon lacerations usually occur during raising of the extensor retinaculum or when the wrist is inadequately exposed resulting in poor protection of the tendons. The tendons most likely to be injured are the digital extensors and those in the first extensor compartment. To protect the tendons of the first extensor compartment, a progressive subperiosteal elevation is performed at the radial styloid as the wrist is flexed to expose the joint. Tendon mobilization is more difficult in a previously operated wrist. To minimize the risk of extensor tendon injury in a previously operated wrist, the tendons are first exposed proximal and distal to the retinaculum. Often the retinaculum is scarred to the overlying skin. In this case, the skin and retinaculum are raised together as radial and ulnar flaps, which also reduces the risk of skin-healing problems.

If a tendon is lacerated it should be repaired using standard techniques. Postoperative rehabilitation is modified slightly to avoid excessive tension on the repair but complete wrist immobilization for an extended period is avoided to prevent wrist stiffness.

Wound Problems

Wound-healing problems are more common in patients with delicate skin but are not unique to patients with rheumatoid arthritis. Other risk factors include the use of steroids for any reason, poorly controlled diabetes, and older age. Hematoma, skin edge necrosis, and wound dehiscence are potential early complications following total wrist arthroplasty. Use of a tourniquet with deflation before closure to obtain hemostasis and use of a closed suction drain for at least 48 hours postoperatively greatly reduces the risk of hematoma. Instructing the patient or family member on how to remove the drain after discharge from the hospital is easy and an effective method to retain the drain. A small hematoma is managed by a gentle compression wrap and delaying the postoperative rehabilitation. Surgical evacuation is considered for a large hematoma.

Use of a local adhesive drape on the skin reduces injury from the instrumentation. Avoiding excessive skin traction is important, especially at the center of the incision when the wrist is flexed. If skin necrosis occurs but is superficial and the wound remains closed, local wound management with moist dressing changes usually suffices. Full digital motion is allowed but the extremes of wrist motion are discouraged until wound healing is nearly complete. Should deep wound dehiscence occur, healing by secondary intention is considered if the area is small and there are no signs of infection. When the defect is large or deep, the best option is surgical debridement and closure with retention-type sutures if this can be accomplished with minimal skin tension. If the defect is too large to close, the wound is prepared and dressed for healing by secondary intention with care to prevent desiccation of the extensor tendons. Only in rare cases would a distant flap be used. A local rotation flap is contraindicated because of the compromised vascularity of the local skin. In general, wound problems should be treated early and aggressively to prevent deep infection.

Extensor Tendon Adhesions

A monitored physical therapy program emphasizing early active and passive digital motion and active wrist motion minimizes the risk of extensor tendon adhesions. If the patient is not able to start early motion because of swelling, pain, wound-healing problems, or concerns with prosthetic instability, then extensor tendon adhesions may develop. Fortunately, tendon gliding and digital motion usually improve with time even without an extensive therapy program. Thus, tenolysis should not be done any sooner than 6 months after surgery. Transposing the tendons superficial to the retinaculum reduces the risk of recurrent adhesions but may create visible prominence beneath the skin. Leaving the tendons subcutaneous at the time of the arthroplasty is also an option in patients who had previous wrist or tendon surgery, however as mentioned earlier, raising the skin and retinaculum together is more advantageous because it is technically easier, causes less skin vascular compromise, and allows single-layer closure that restores the retinaculum.

Wrist Stiffness

Of concern to the patient is wrist stiffness because arthroplasty was selected over arthrodesis to retain motion. Although range of motion varies slightly among available implants, all designs provide a functional range of motion albeit not normal. Early stiffness often improves with time and returning to activities, with maximum motion not expected until 6 months. However, if a gradual improvement is not seen after the second month, then a more regular therapy program is initiated. Passive motion exercises, intermittent dynamic

splinting, and static night splinting are included in the program.

In rare cases, surgery can be attempted to improve motion. To improve flexion, an extensor tenolysis and dorsal capsular slide are considered, whereas extension may require flexor tendon step-cut lengthening (flexor carpi ulnaris [FCU] and flexor carpi radialis [FCR]) and volar capsular slide. A capsular slide is done by raising it as a distally based flap in continuity with the distal 1 cm of the periosteum over the radius. The wrist is then flexed or extended, which causes the capsule to slide distally. The new edge of the capsule is sutured to the rim of the radius. If there is insufficient capsule length for a slide, an allograft (tensor fascia lata is my preference) is used to bridge between the proximal edge of the capsule and the rim of the radius. The wrist is immobilized in the improved position for a short time followed by regular therapy and splinting.

Wrist Imbalance

Wrist imbalance was common for ball-and-socket and hinge designs. The wrist would typically fall into ulnar deviation and often flexion.[6,16] Newer designs with a broad articulation in the radioulnar dimension have greatly reduced imbalance but it can still be a challenging problem in patients with deformed and contracted wrists preoperatively. Accurate implant alignment and proper tensioning of the capsule and tendons are keys to attaining good motion and balance. Although imbalance may occasionally correct with time and with postoperative splinting, it should not be expected to do so, and in fact there is a substantial risk the deformity will increase. Thus, it is much more effective and reliable to recognize and correct imbalance at the time of surgery. Patients with juvenile rheumatoid arthritis are particularly difficult cases because of the combination of bone erosion and flexor tendon tightness. During the initial surgery, imbalance may respond to 1 or a combination of simple maneuvers such as changing the polyethylene bearing thickness, an additional resection of the distal radius to reduce volar capsule tension, or flexor tendon lengthening. Most frequently the FCU is lengthened, however, lengthening the FCR may occasionally be necessary. In patients with volar wrist subluxation, the distal radius has often been remodeled to create a large volar extension from the edge of the lunate fossa. This excess bone must be removed to avoid tightness of the capsule and a volar prominence once the wrist is reduced with the implant.

These techniques can also be used during revision surgery if the imbalance did not respond to time and conservative measures. Component revision or conversion to an arthrodesis are the only options if postoperative imbalance is caused by improperly positioned components.

Distal Radioulnar Joint Problems

Management of the distal radioulnar joint (DRUJ) implant at the time of the initial wrist arthroplasty depends on the status of its articular surfaces, its alignment, the type of disease, and most important, whether it is symptomatic. Sometimes it is difficult to determine if an arthritic DRUJ is contributing to the symptoms, in which case 1 option is to leave the DRUJ intact but advise the patient that further surgery may be necessary. Preserving the ulnar head is particularly considered for patients with posttraumatic or osteoarthritis in whom the DRUJ is nearly free of arthritis and ulnar variance is neutral or negative. Modification of the wrist arthroplasty technique may be required, including free-hand cutting, to ensure the sigmoid notch and DRUJ are preserved.

Surgical options include complete excision of the head, synovectomy alone, hemiresection arthroplasty, and implant arthroplasty. Patients with rheumatoid arthritis are usually best treated by complete ulnar head excision even if there is minimal arthritic involvement because of the possibility of developing symptomatic arthritis of the DRUJ and the low incidence of complaints related to excision in this population (**Fig. 3**). The young patient with rheumatoid arthritis with oligoarticular disease and minimal erosions may be a candidate for synovectomy alone and preserving the ulnar head, however excision at some future time should be anticipated. Complete ulnar head excision is also indicated when there is substantial radiocarpal articular destruction resulting in loss of wrist height and positive ulnar variance. In this situation, preparation of the radius will remove too much of the sigmoid notch for the DRUJ to remain functional. Although hemiresection arthroplasty of the distal ulna is an option, impingement between the ulnar styloid and the carpal component may occur. This procedure is best indicated for patients with posttraumatic or osteoarthritis in whom the radiocarpal height is relatively well preserved and the DRUJ is arthritic. Precise contouring of the head and adequate soft tissue interposition between the radius and ulna are keys to a successful result.

Many patients experience radioulnar impingement with crepitance after complete ulnar head excision is performed. Concomitant stabilization

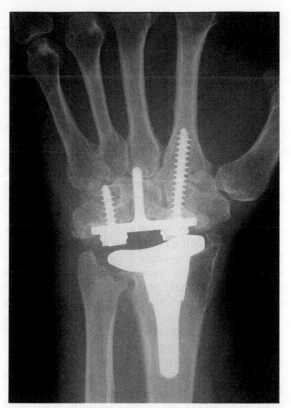

Fig. 3. DRUJ symptomatic arthritis developed in a patient with rheumatoid arthritis treated initially with a UNI 2 implant and retention of the distal ulna. A secondary Darrach procedure relieved the symptoms.

procedures do not seem to affect the incidence. Symptoms are typically mild and usually resolve in a few months. A pseudo-articulation with scalloping of the radius may develop but this usually stabilizes by the first year and is not symptomatic. Some patients in whom the DRUJ was retained may go on to develop symptomatic arthritis. Treatment is excision of the ulnar head through a second ulnar incision directly over the head and closure of the capsule without a specific stabilization procedure unless gross instability is noted. In rare cases, instability of the ulna stump remains symptomatic following a primary or secondary excision. Soft tissue interposition with a stabilization procedure using extensor carpi ulnaris or FCU is most commonly used to mitigate symptoms of impingement.

Although combined total wrist and DRUJ implant arthroplasty has been used, the results are still preliminary and there is concern that metal on metal wear may develop if there is progressive sigmoid notch erosion caused by the ulnar implant.

Prosthetic Instability

Early postoperative prosthetic dislocation is usually caused by soft tissue imbalance or excessive joint laxity. Patients with rheumatoid arthritis with longstanding wrist deformity and severe active synovitis are at greatest risk. Loss of bone stock decreases the overall length of the wrist and chronic synovitis causes attenuation of the wrist capsule and weakening of the muscles resulting in joint subluxation. Patients with substantial active synovitis or inadequate bone stock because of skeletal erosions are poor candidates for arthroplasty, however patients with deficient wrist capsule alone can be augmented with allograft tissue (tensor fascia lata) to provide stability and coverage of the prosthesis (**Fig. 4**). Early instability is treated by casting the wrist in its most stable position for several weeks to allow the capsule to heal and tighten. Secondary allograft capsule augmentation and tendon rebalancing is a feasible treatment of early and late instability unresponsive to conservative measures, however soft tissue procedures will not rescue a malaligned, improperly implanted prosthesis.

Late or recurrent prosthetic instability may be caused by gradual attenuation of the capsule or poor component alignment. Designs with small contact areas have a higher risk of instability and dislocation. An articulation with broader contact area throughout its range of motion provides greater prosthetic stability and allows early postoperative motion without reducing total final motion. Treatment of late prosthetic instability or dislocation does not usually respond permanently to immobilization alone unless there was an acute event, and instability is typically difficult to treat surgically because component revision can be destructive to the skeleton. Hence, the potential major contributing factors of instability should be identified as best possible before undertaking revision surgery. Component alignment is critically assessed on true posterior-anterior and lateral radiographs and, if necessary, in positions of prosthetic instability. If recent trauma contributed to the instability, a trial of immobilization is attempted. An external fixator that spans the wrist and implant has been used successfully to treat recurrent instability (**Fig. 5**). If component alignment is satisfactory and there is no active synovitis, secondary capsule reconstruction using allograft is an option. Prosthetic systems with modular designs may respond to increasing the polyethylene bearing thickness, however the capsule must be intact or reconstructed for this method to be effective long-term, as increasing the bearing width may otherwise increase instability. When the capsule seems adequate and the tendons well balanced, an option is revision to a more stable design or conversion to an arthrodesis. Techniques for revision arthroplasty are described later.

Implant Loosening

Historically, implant loosening was common, especially of carpal components fixed into the metacarpal shafts.[6–8,16] Newer designs are fixed to the carpus and incorporate an intercarpal arthrodesis, which improves support for the carpal component and reduces loosening.[11] However, exuberant synovitis, poor bone stock, and the use of the upper extremities for ambulation contribute substantially to aseptic implant loosening. Patient selection and education are the keys to reduce these risks. All patients should be cautioned against forceful repetitive use of the wrist after arthroplasty. Yearly follow-up radiographs are recommended to monitor for subsidence or loosening of the components. Mild subsidence often stabilizes and does not require intervention, however progressive subsidence should not be ignored even if the patient is

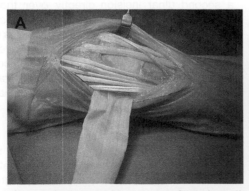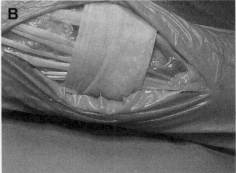

Fig. 4. Wrist implant covered by a tensor fascia lata allograft (A) because of extremely poor capsule tissue from disease and previous surgery. Graft was then folded back to reconstruct the extensor retinaculum (B).

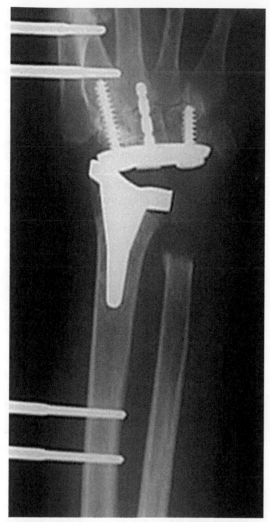

Fig. 5. A spanning external fixator has been used successfully in select cases of instability that cannot be controlled by casting after a traumatic episode. Note that excessive resection of the distal ulna likely contributed to the instability.

be made over the dorsal midline of the radius, because this would interfere with plate and screw application. A similar technique can be used to remove a distal component fixed in a metacarpal shaft. Circumferential cerclage wires are used to restore structural integrity to the bone. Cortical strut grafts are used if necessary for extensive bone loss but excessive bulk may make skin closure tight. If a revision arthroplasty is performed, I prefer cement fixation, especially if there is substantial bone loss. Impaction grafting techniques can be used if the cortex is severely thinned but extensive grafting for bone loss is unreliable. A minimum of 50% of the capitate height is necessary for a revision arthroplasty. In revision arthroplasty, the CMC joints should be formally fused if any portion of the implant or screws crosses a joint.

When there is substantial bone loss that would result in questionable component fixation or the patient has been excessively active, then conversion to an arthrodesis is the best option.[17,18] Because there is typically substantial bone loss when converting to a fusion, a structural bone graft is necessary and plate fixation for long-term rigidity is preferable. One study found the use of femoral head allograft to be equal to iliac crest autograft in achieving fusion and without the obvious drawbacks of harvesting iliac crest (**Fig. 6**).[19] I prefer to use only the cancellous portion of the femoral head allograft, to size it to restore wrist height, and to shape it to fit all of the defects in the radius and carpus, that is, the distal canal of the radius and the erosions in the carpus. A typically wrist arthrodesis plate is applied. Because graft incorporation requires several months, the wrist should be splinted until radiographic healing is evident to reduce the risk of plate loosening and nonunion.

asymptomatic as revision surgery becomes much more difficult with carpus erosion. Treatment of a loose implant depends primarily on the remaining bone stock but in generally conversion to a fusion is the preferred option. If there is adequate bone stock, especially of the carpus, and all other factors are also positive, then revision arthroplasty is an acceptable option.

Removal of implants for revision arthroplasty or conversion to a complete wrist fusion can be difficult if the components are well fixed, especially if cement was used. A dorsal-radial osteotomy of the radius followed by gently prying open the cortex allows access to the cement and reduces the risk of creating a more serious, uncontrolled fracture of the radius. The osteotomy should not

Infection

Infection is an infrequent but serious complication. An attempt to salvage an early postoperative infection by surgical debridement is indicated for gram-positive organisms with sufficient sensitivity to antibiotics. A late infection is best treated with resection arthroplasty and delayed complete wrist arthrodesis once the organism is identified and an appropriate antibiotic treatment is completed, as well as a period of time free of treatment and infection. Antibiotic impregnated cement spacer or beads are typically used as an adjunct to intravenous antibiotics and to maintain wrist height until a fusion is performed. Repeated debridement with a new antibiotic spacer or beads may be required.

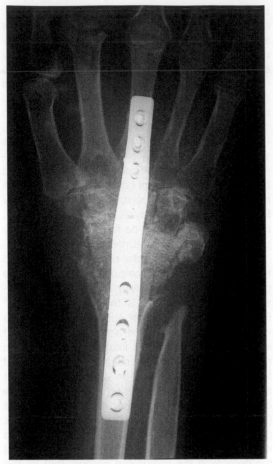

Fig. 6. Loose wrist implant treated by femoral head allograft and dorsal arthrodesis plate.

SUMMARY

Total wrist arthroplasty is a valuable option in the treatment of severe wrist arthritis if the patient's activity demands and wrist condition are appropriate. Wound problems, joint imbalance and instability, implant loosening, DRUJ problems, tendon adhesions, and infection can occur. Awareness of potential complications, careful patient selection, thorough preoperative planning, and precise surgical technique minimize these risks. Proper early management also reduces the morbidity caused by complications. Although most complications are treatable, conversion to a complete arthrodesis may be necessary and fortunately is more reliable and causes less morbidity than fusion of other major joints.

REFERENCES

1. Vicar AJ, Burton RI. Surgical management of the rheumatoid wrist fusion or arthroplasty. J Hand Surg Am 1986;11(6):790–7.

2. Swanson AB. Flexible implant arthroplasty for arthritic disabilities of the radiocarpal joint. A silicone rubber intramedullary stemmed flexible hinge implant for the wrist joint. Orthop Clin North Am 1973;4(2):383–94.

3. Jolly SL, Ferlic DC, Clayton ML, et al. Swanson silicone arthroplasty of the wrist in rheumatoid arthritis: a long-term follow-up. J Hand Surg Am 1992;17(1): 142–9.

4. Peimer CA, Medige J, Eckert BS, et al. Reactive synovitis after silicone arthroplasty. J Hand Surg Am 1986;11(5):624–38.

5. Ferlic DC, Jolly SN, Clayton ML. Salvage for failed implant arthroplasty of the wrist. J Hand Surg Am 1992;17(5):917–23.

6. Meuli HC. Total wrist arthroplasty. Experience with a noncemented wrist prosthesis. Clin Orthop 1997; 342:77–83.

7. Dennis DA, Ferlic DC, Clayton ML. Volz total wrist arthroplasty in rheumatoid arthritis: a long-term review. J Hand Surg Am 1986;11(4):483–90.

8. Menon J. Total wrist replacement using the modified Volz prosthesis. J Bone Joint Surg Am 1987;69(7): 998–1006.

9. Figgie MP, Ranawat CS, Inglis AE, et al. Trispherical total wrist arthroplasty in rheumatoid arthritis. J Hand Surg Am 1990;15(2):217–23.

10. Cobb TK, Beckenbaugh RD. Biaxial total-wrist arthroplasty. J Hand Surg Am 1996;21(6):1011–21.

11. Cobb TK, Beckenbaugh RD. Biaxial long-stemmed multipronged distal components for revision/bone deficit total-wrist arthroplasty. J Hand Surg Am 1996;21(5):764–70.

12. Radmer S, Andresen R, Sparmann M. Wrist arthroplasty with a new generation of prostheses in patients with rheumatoid arthritis. J Hand Surg Am 1999;24(5):935–43.

13. Menon J. Universal total wrist implant: experience with a carpal component fixed with 3 screws. J Arthroplasty 1998;13(5):515–23.

14. Grosland NM, Rogge RD, Adams BD. Influence of arthicular geometry on prosthetic wrist stability. Clin Orthop 2004;421:134–42.

15. Divelbiss BJ, Sollerman C, Adams BD. Early results of the Universal total wrist arthroplasty in rheumatoid arthritis. J Hand Surg Am 2002;27(2):195–204.

16. Lorei MP, Figgie MP, Ranawat CS, et al. Failed total wrist arthroplasty. Analysis of failures and results of operative management. Clin Orthop 1997;342:84–93.

17. Cooney WP 3rd, Beckenbaugh RD, Linscheid RL. Total wrist arthroplasty. Problems with implant failures. Clin Orthop 1984;187:121–8.

18. Adams BD. Total wrist arthroplasty. Semin Arthroplasty 2000;11:72–81.

19. Carloon JR, Simmono BP. Total wrist arthroplasty. J Am Acad Orthop Surg 1998;6(5):308–15.

Complications of Limited and Total Wrist Arthrodesis

Robert W. Wysocki, MD[a,b,*], Mark S. Cohen, MD[a,b]

KEYWORDS

- Total wrist arthrodesis • Partial wrist arthrodesis
- Complications • Four-corner fusion

Partial and total wrist arthrodeses have become common procedures for treating degenerative diseases arising from numerous conditions, including posttraumatic arthrosis, intercalated segment instability, inflammatory arthropathy, and carpal osteonecrosis. Wrist arthrodesis also has a role in the treatment of midcarpal instability, severe spastic deformity, paralysis of the hand, and bone loss from tumor or trauma. The first report of total wrist arthrodesis dates back to 1910 in treatment of tuberculosis,[1] and Thornton[2] reported on the first limited wrist fusion in 1924 when he successfully fused the scaphoid, lunate, capitate, and hamate.

The goals of limited wrist arthrodesis are similar to those of total wrist arthrodesis in providing pain relief and improved function by fusing across arthritic or unstable joints, with the added benefit of motion preservation. Biomechanical studies have determined that between 30% and 50% of sagittal motion at the wrist occurs through the midcarpal joint, with the remainder through the radiocarpal joint.[3,4] Sparing of either the midcarpal or the radiocarpal articulations avoids complete loss of wrist motion, and a compensatory increase in motion at the unfused joint has been shown for up to 1 year postoperatively.[5,6] Despite the success, wrist arthrodeses are not without risk, and overall minor and major complication rates of up to 51% to 68% have been reported in large series.[7,8] Awareness of the complications associated with wrist arthrodesis and how best to avoid them is essential for the treating physician to appropriately counsel patients on different arthrodesis options and to inform them on what to expect from the procedure.

Although many different versions of wrist arthrodesis have been described, this article focuses on the complications associated with total wrist fusion and the more common limited arthrodeses, including scaphoid excision and four-corner fusion, scaphotrapeziotrapezoid (STT) fusion, and isolated radiocarpal fusion.

NONUNION

Nonunion after wrist arthrodesis is directly related to several factors. The first is the articulations of the individual bones within the carpus. The size of the bones and the small surface area of the joints would appear set up for nonunion, especially in comparison with the large torques that are applied to the carpal bones by the intrinsic and extrinsic ligaments of the wrist. This has been corroborated by the poor fusion rates in attempts at arthrodesis of single articulations within the carpus, including the scapholunate[9,10] and lunotriquetral[10,11] joints (**Fig. 1**). It is for this reason that adjacent carpal bones are now included in limited fusions, such as STT fusion and four-corner fusion, which show improved union rates without established deleterious effects (**Fig. 2**).[12] The second important factor for achieving union is the stability of fixation. Total wrist arthrodesis evolved over

a Department of Orthopaedic Surgery, Rush University, Chicago, IL, USA
b Midwest Orthopaedics at Rush, 1611 West Harrison Street, Suite 400, Chicago, IL 60612, USA
* Corresponding author. Midwest Orthopaedics at Rush, 1611 West Harrison Street, Suite 400, Chicago, IL 60612.
E-mail address: robertwysocki@mac.com

Hand Clin 26 (2010) 221–228
doi:10.1016/j.hcl.2009.11.003

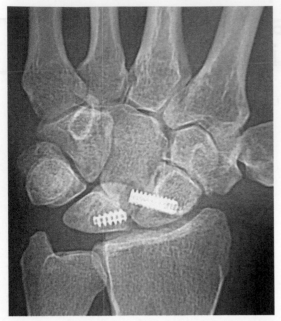

Fig. 1. Anteroposterior radiograph showing failed arthrodesis of the scapholunate joint with a broken compression screw.

time from uninstrumented fusion with structural corticocancellous graft,[13] to transarticular pin fixation,[14] to intramedullary fixation,[15] and most recently to dorsal compression plating,[8,10,16] which has achieved nonunion rates of 2% to 4%[8,16] as opposed to rates as high as 19%[17] by using older fixation techniques. Hastings and colleagues,[8] in their series of 90 wrists, noted a nonunion rate of 2% with dorsal plating compared with 18% with other techniques. Although limited wrist arthrodesis has traditionally been performed with pin fixation, the use of circular plates with the theoretical advantage of increased construct rigidity gained popularity in the past, especially for scaphoid excision and four-corner fusion. However, although comprehensive literature reviews covering decades of treatment have reported nonunion rates between 4% and 8% in four-corner fusions with pin fixation,[10,18,19] the union results with circular plate fixation have been much more variable, with nonunion rates as high as 10% to 62.5%.[20–23] The initial enthusiasm for these has now waned.

Several other factors that affect union after wrist arthrodesis must be considered irrespective of the fixation type or site of fusion. Preparation of the fusion surfaces is critical and must include meticulous removal of all articular cartilages (**Fig. 3**A) and direct apposition of the surfaces, with compression when possible at the time of application of fixation. Compression specifically improves stability. The use and type of bone graft used are also potential factors. Although there is no good comparative data specifically addressing bone graft in this setting, it has been our experience that the excised carpal bones are often sclerotic with minimal good-quality cancellous bone, and thus we advocate the use of distal radius, iliac crest, or other source of fresh cancellous autograft packed into the fusion surfaces (**Fig. 3**B). Patient-related factors, such as avoiding tobacco use and compliance with immobilization and activity restriction until union are critical, and their importance must be communicated to the patient.

In comparison to total wrist arthrodesis and four-corner fusion, the nonunion rates of other common wrist arthrodeses seem higher. Series of STT fusions have had nonunion rates ranging from 0% to 29%,[24–28] with a meta-analysis reporting 14% nonunion.[10] Watson and colleagues[25] reported a nonunion rate of 4% in their large series of 800 STT fusions, well below most other rates in the literature, and these authors emphasize generous preparation of the fusion bed by resecting more than just the articular surface to provide well-opposed edges, routine use of distal radius cancellous autograft, parallel pins to allow compression along the pin axis, and 3 weeks of long-arm immobilization including the thumb followed by short-arm immobilization. Nonunion rates are less frequently reported after radioscapholunate fusion and vary from 5% to 27%.[29–31]

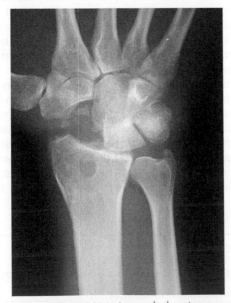

Fig. 2. Anteroposterior radiograph showing a successful scaphoid excision and four-corner fusion.

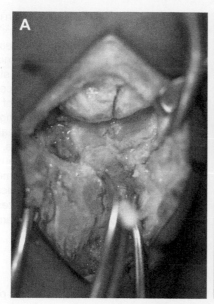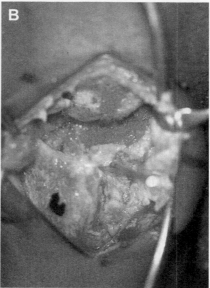

Fig. 3. The fusion surfaces after (*A*) removal of the articular cartilage and (*B*) placement of cancellous autograft during the preparation for scaphoid excision and four-corner fusion.

INFECTION AND WOUND COMPLICATIONS

Several aspects of wrist arthrodeses make these procedures prone to wound complications. The exposure often requires raising large soft-tissue flaps and the dorsal wrist skin, and subcutaneous tissue can be thin, especially in patients with inflammatory arthropathy who have been on oral steroid therapy. The extensive bony preparation required also predisposes patients to postoperative hematoma formation.

Overall wound complication rates associated with partial and total wrist fusions, including blistering, hematoma, and minor dehiscence, have been reported in 20% to 30% of cases.[7,8,17] Most tend to resolve without reoperation, although complete wound breakdown requiring secondary skin grafting has been reported.[32] Infection rates seem to be low, with a superficial infection rate of about 3% and a deep infection rate of 0.5%.[7,8,17,19,33,34]

Several steps can be taken to reduce the likelihood of wound complications. Preoperatively, appropriately administered prophylactic antibiotics against typical skin pathogens are routinely used. Intraoperatively, full-thickness flaps down to retinaculum and meticulous hemostasis are especially important. Postoperatively, a compressive dressing and a temporary splint may help soft-tissue healing.

HARDWARE COMPLICATIONS

The thin nature of the skin and the subcutaneous tissue of the dorsal wrist that predisposes to wound complications predisposes patients to symptomatic prominent hardware. Dorsal compression plating with a small fragment implant has resulted in symptomatic hardware in the form of either a painful prominence or a bursa in 35% to 65% of cases,[32,35–37] frequently requiring implant removal (**Fig. 4**). Although there is no universally agreed upon standard, plate removal should not be attempted until 6 months and preferably 12 months after placement, with clear evidence of radiographic union.

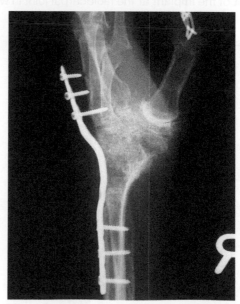

Fig. 4. Lateral radiograph after total wrist arthrodesis showing pullout of the dorsal plate.

Removal of the implant is not without consequence, as fractures through previous screw holes in the radius[32] and in the metacarpal[7,8] requiring replating have been reported. Immobilization of the wrist and limited activity for 6 weeks after implant removal should be strongly considered.

Extensor tendon adhesions and synovitis are also not uncommon after total wrist arthrodesis, likely from a combination of irritation over a dorsal implant and postoperative scarring. The need for repeat operation for tenosynovectomy and tenolysis has been reported to be as high as 43%, with dorsal plate fixation in total wrist fusion.[8] Intraoperatively, at the time of arthrodesis, all attempts should be made at interposing tissue between hardware and the extensor tendons. It is helpful to elevate the fourth dorsal compartment subperiosteally, maintaining the subsheath around the tendons for protection. If the joint capsule is insufficient to cover a small area of hardware, a transverse incision across the retinaculum can allow one half of the retinaculum to be placed between the plate and the tendons and the other half to be repaired to its normal position to prevent bowstringing. Early range of motion of the digits postoperatively and attention to this potential complication during physiotherapy is critical. The use of newer precontoured total wrist fusion plates that have a smaller dimension over the metacarpal than traditional small fragment implants have shown promising results in decreasing the rate of hardware-related complications.[38,39]

Circular plate fixation for scaphoid excision and four-corner fusion carries a risk of dorsal impingement of the implant at the radiocarpal joint in wrist extension (**Fig. 5**A). This is reported in up to 22% of cases by Vance and colleagues[22] and 25% of cases by Shindle and colleagues.[23] The site of fixation must be adequately reamed such that the implant will sit flush with or even slightly buried below the dorsal articular surface (**Fig. 5**B). Maximal bone stock and length of the carpus must be preserved while preparing the fusion surfaces so that the plate's proximal edge does not end up too close to the radius. It is critical that the lunate be reduced into neutral or slight flexion to restore midcarpal alignment (**Fig. 6**). This not only optimizes biomechanics to provide wrist extension[40] but also maximizes the length of the carpus to provide more clearance for the implant.

NERVE COMPLICATIONS

Injury to the major peripheral nerves of the hand is an uncommon complication of wrist arthrodesis,[7] as they are usually located away from the surgical site during a dorsal approach. Dorsal sensory branches of the radial and ulnar nerves, conversely, are more at risk during wrist arthrodesis from injury during the surgical dissection and the placement of percutaneous pins. Reported rates of either painful neuroma or decreased sensation in a sensory nerve distribution most commonly range between 2% and 5%,[7,8,22,32,35,41,42] and it is not clearly established if the risk is higher with plate or percutaneous pin fixation.[8,22] To help prevent these complications during open dorsal exposures, sensory branches should be kept in the flaps and protected from

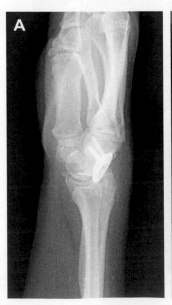
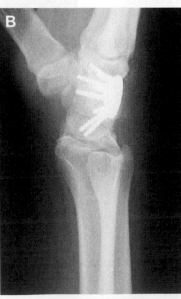

Fig. 5. Lateral radiographs after scaphoid excision and four-corner fusion showing (*A*) an extended lunate and dorsal prominence of the plate leading to impingement and (*B*) a correctly positioned lunate and well-seated plate with no dorsal impingement.

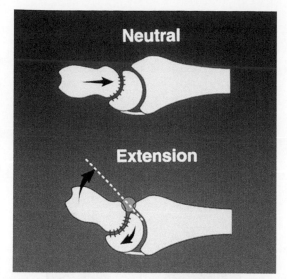

Fig. 6. Dorsal impingement secondary to an extended lunate compared with neutral alignment.

excessive retraction throughout the procedure. If pin fixation is going to be used outside the dorsal incision, we recommend wires be placed either percutaneously through a 16-gauge needle as a soft-tissue protector or under direct visualization through a small open incision. This is especially critical on the radial side of the wrist in the area of the dorsal sensory radial nerve branches.

Postoperative carpal tunnel syndrome is a well-recognized complication of total wrist arthrodesis. This complication is reported less frequently with limited wrist arthrodesis. The incidence seems higher with dorsal plate fixation than with other means,[8] with an overall rate of 10% to 25% after plate fixation. Approximately half of these cases require carpal tunnel release eventually.[8,17,36] We routinely perform a carpal tunnel release with total wrist arthrodesis to avoid this complication.

Complex regional pain syndrome is a rare but devastating complication of wrist arthrodesis, with a reported incidence of approximately 2% to 3% in larger series.[8,19,32] Rates are similar between total and limited wrist fusions. Avoidance of tight dressings; adequate pain control; and early recognition and treatment of dystrophic signs and symptoms with appropriate physiotherapy and agents such as calcium channel blockers, oral steroids, and neuroactive agents have roles in prevention and treatment. If early symptoms progress, consultation from a pain specialist is often warranted with a multidisciplinary approach to the condition.

ADJACENT ARTHRITIS

Degenerative disease in adjacent joints has been reported in the distal radioulnar joint (DRUJ) after total arthrodesis. Symptomatic DRUJ arthritis that required distal ulna resection in 3% of patients at a mean period of 1 year has been reported in one series.[7] Adjacent arthritis is more common after limited wrist arthrodesis (**Fig. 7**), with radiocarpal and trapeziometacarpal arthritis reported in long-term series of STT fusions. At 5 years postoperatively, Fortin and Louis[26] found adjacent

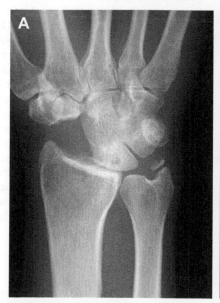
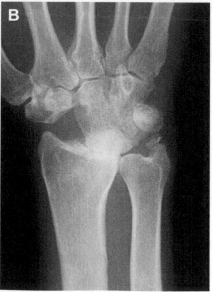

Fig. 7. Anteroposterior radiographs after scaphoid excision and four-corner fusion (*A*) at the time of radiographic arthrodesis and (*B*) 5 years postoperatively showing advanced adjacent arthritis of the radiolunate joint.

degenerative disease in 71% of their cohort, with inadequate reduction of the scaphoid being predictive for a poor outcome. Series by Minami and colleagues[24] and Kleinman[43] have reported incidences of 23% and 19%, respectively. Secondary midcarpal arthrosis after radioscapholunate arthrodesis occurs in approximately one-third of patients in long-term follow-up, and the rates were similar whether the procedure was done for posttraumatic arthrosis or inflammatory arthropathy.[30,44,45] Patients must be carefully screened and selected, as preexisting adjacent joint arthrosis may preclude limited arthrodesis. In limited arthrodeses that preserve the radioscaphoid articulation, it is critical that the scaphoid be reduced into as anatomic a position as possible, given its complex shape.[26,43] Conversely, the relatively uniform convexity of the lunate's articular surface with the radius likely explains the paucity of radiolunate arthrosis that occurs after scaphoid excision and four-corner fusion.

IMPACTION

Total wrist arthrodesis has been associated with ulnocarpal abutment, which manifests as ulnar wrist pain caused by forearm rotation activities of daily living or firm gripping or grasping.[7] Patients whose fixation extends onto the second metacarpal instead of the third may be positioned in an additional ulnar deviation that may predispose to abutment. An incidence for this complication is difficult to estimate. Zachary and Stern[7] reported one case in their series (with an overall incidence of 1%) that was treated with a distal ulna resection, and Trumble and colleagues[46] reported on a series of 3 cases, all of which had good results from excision of the pisiform or triquetrum. This complication, when recognized, is best treated with joint leveling procedures in ulnar positive patients, especially if they are young and the DRUJ is intact. Resection of either the distal ulna or the diseased portions of the carpus is recommended in older lower-demand patients with ulnar neutral or negative variance or an unsalvageable DRUJ.

IMPINGEMENT

Radial styloid impingement is a well-recognized complication of STT fusion. Rogers and Watson reported this complication in 33% of their original series of 93 patients, with 18% requiring a secondary radial styloidectomy. They recommended routine styloidectomy as an integral component of an STT fusion (**Fig. 8**).[47] Watson and Wollstein[19] later reported an improved secondary radial styloidectomy rate of 7.3%,

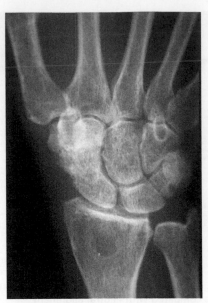

Fig. 8. Anteroposterior radiograph of a successfully fused STT arthrodesis with radial styloidectomy.

performed at 1.2 years postoperatively in their follow-up series of 800 STT fusions. They noted a higher incidence of radial styloid impingement in patients treated for scapholunate ligament injury than those treated for Kienbock disease. Because other preferred treatment options exist for scapholunate ligament injury and Kienbock disease, we believe that the principle indication for STT fusion is for isolated STT arthritis. We support Watson and Wollstein's recommendation of routine radial styloidectomy. Reduction of the extended scaphoid to a position of neutral or slight volar flexion within the scaphoid fossa is critically emphasized.[48] The irregular shape of the scaphoid coupled with its frequently extended position preoperatively serve as explanations for the higher rates of impingement in patients with the abnormal kinematics of scapholunate ligament injury.

The rates of dorsal impingement after scaphoid excision and four-corner fusion with traditional fixation techniques after comprehensive review are reported as 4%.[19] Early reports of the rate of impingement with dorsal circular plating are variable but seem higher than with traditional methods. The most important technical aspect of this procedure to avoid impingement involves proper rotation and reduction of the lunate as discussed earlier (see **Fig. 6**).

PERSISTENT PAIN

Despite the theoretical benefit of eliminating pain via fusion of diseased articulations, wrist arthrodesis does have significant rates of persistent pain associated with it, especially after activity and heavy work. The ability to draw conclusions from the literature regarding persistent pain is limited by the different ways in which investigators measure and describe impairment. For total wrist arthrodesis, Sauerbier and colleagues[49] found that 70% of patients had no pain at rest, but only 40% had no pain with work or heavy use. De Smet and Truyen's results were somewhat worse, reporting that 55% of patients were pain-free at rest and only 17% were pain-free with manual activity.[50] Zachary and Stern reported significant chronic pain in 8% of their series.[7]

Tomaino and colleagues[51] and Wyrick and colleagues[52] looked specifically at persistent pain after scaphoid excision and four-corner fusion and found more than 25% of patients with scaphoid excision and four-corner fusion to have either severe persistent pain or inadequate pain relief. Vance and colleagues[22] reported moderate or severe pain in 53% of patients after plate fixation and 21% after pin fixation for four-corner fusion. More promising results have been shown by Cohen and Kozin[40] who showed that 21% of patients have long-term requirement for pain medicine, and Merrell and colleagues[33] who found a mean Visual Analog Scale pain score of 2.3 and an 88% return to manual labor. Few series of STT or limited radiocarpal fusions have reported on generalized persistent pain, with most focusing on the onset of radiographically proven adjacent arthritis, the results of which have already been discussed.

Although it is difficult to reach definitive conclusions regarding pain relief based on the existing data, it must be stressed that during the preoperative evaluation, all potential sites of arthrosis within the wrist and carpus must be closely assessed radiographically and by direct inspection, so that an inadequate or an inappropriate procedure does not fail early because of the development of early adjacent arthritis. As for generalized persistent pain, it is fair to warn patients, especially those who are higher-demand individuals, that although most series agree that patients improve from their preoperative condition, it is not uncommon to have persistent pain especially with activity. This is especially true in total wrist arthrodesis in higher-demand individuals.

SUMMARY

Total and partial wrist arthrodeses encompass various procedures to treat numerous conditions. It is this variability that mandates meticulous preoperative consideration of each patient's specific pathology and goals. Despite the high overall minor and major complication rates frequently reported with wrist arthrodesis, most of these tend to be temporary and do not preclude a good outcome. A thorough understanding of the complications and the best practices to avoid them is critical for the surgeon in the preoperative, intraoperative, and postoperative management of candidates for total or limited wrist arthrodesis.

REFERENCES

1. Ely LW. A study of joint tuberculosis. Surg Gynecol Obstet 1910;10:561–72.
2. Thornton L. Old dislocation of os magnum: open reduction and stabilization. South Med J 1924;17:430.
3. Gellman H, Kauffman D, Lenihan M, et al. An in vitro analysis of wrist motion: the effect of limited intercarpal arthrodesis and the contributions of the radiocarpal and midcarpal joints. J Hand Surg Am 1988;13: 378–83.
4. Wolfe SW, Neu C, Crisco JJ. In vivo scaphoid, lunate, and capitate kinematics in flexion and in extension. J Hand Surg Am 2000;25:860–9.
5. Watson HK, Goodman ML, Johnson TR. Limited wrist arthrodesis. Part II: intercarpal and radiocarpal combinations. J Hand Surg Am 1981;6:223–33.
6. Watson HK, Hempton RF. Limited wrist arthrodeses. I. The triscaphoid joint. J Hand Surg Am 1980;5:320–7.
7. Zachary SV, Stern PJ. Complications following AO/ASIF wrist arthrodesis. J Hand Surg Am 1995;20:339–44.
8. Hastings H II, Weiss AP, Quenzer D, et al. Arthrodesis of the wrist for post-traumatic disorders. J Bone Joint Surg Am 1996;78:897–902.
9. Hom S, Ruby LK. Attempted scapholunate arthrodesis for chronic scapholunate dissociation. J Hand Surg Am 1991;16:334–9.
10. Larsen CF, Jacoby RA, McCabe SJ. Nonunion rates of limited carpal arthrodesis: a meta-analysis of the literature. J Hand Surg Am 1997;22:66–73.
11. Vandesande W, De Smet L, Van Ransbeeck H. Lunotriquetral arthrodesis, a procedure with a high failure rate. Acta Orthop Belg 2001;67:361–7.
12. Krakauer JD, Bishop AT, Cooney WP. Surgical treatment of scapholunate advanced collapse. J Hand Surg Am 1994;19:751–9.
13. Evans DL. Wedge arthrodesis of the wrist. J Bone Joint Surg Br 1955;37:126–34.
14. Campbell CJ, Keokarn T. Total and subtotal arthrodesis of the wrist. J Bone Joint Surg Am 1964;46: 1520–33.
15. Mannerfelt L, Malmsten M. Arthrodesis of the wrist in rheumatoid arthritis. A technique without external fixation. Scand J Plast Reconstr Surg 1971;5:124–30.
16. Wright CS, McMurtry RY. AO arthrodesis in the hand. J Hand Surg Am 1983;8:932–5.
17. Clendenin MB, Green DP. Arthrodesis of the wrist-complications and their management. J Hand Surg Am 1981;6:253–7.

18. Siegel JM, Ruby LK. A critical look at intercarpal arthrodesis: review of the literature. J Hand Surg Am 1996;21:717–23.

19. Shin AY. Four-corner arthrodesis. J Am Soc Surg Hand 2001;1:93–111.

20. Chung KC, Watt AJ, Kotsis SV. A prospective outcomes study of four-corner wrist arthrodesis using a circular limited wrist fusion plate for stage II scapholunate advanced collapse wrist deformity. Plast Reconstr Surg 2006;118:433–42.

21. Kendall CB, Brown TR, Millon SJ, et al. Results of four-corner arthrodesis using dorsal circular plate fixation. J Hand Surg Am 2005;30:903–7.

22. Vance MC, Hernandez JD, Didonna ML, et al. Complications and outcome of four-corner arthrodesis: circular plate fixation versus traditional techniques. J Hand Surg Am 2005;30:1122–7.

23. Shindle MK, Burton KJ, Weiland AJ, et al. Complications of circular plate fixation for four-corner arthrodesis. J Hand Surg Eur Vol 2007;32:50–3.

24. Minami A, Kato H, Suenaga N, et al. Scaphotrapeziotrapezoid fusion: long-term follow-up study. J Orthop Sci 2003;8:319–22.

25. Watson HK, Wollstein R, Joseph E, et al. Scaphotrapeziotrapezoid arthrodesis: a follow-up study. J Hand Surg Am 2003;28:397–404.

26. Fortin PT, Louis DS. Long-term follow-up of scaphoid-trapezium-trapezoid arthrodesis. J Hand Surg Am 1993;18:675–81.

27. McAuliffe JA, Dell PC, Jaffe R. Complications of intercarpal arthrodesis. J Hand Surg Am 1993;18:1121–8.

28. Frykman EB, Af Ekenstam F, Wadin K. Triscaphoid arthrodesis and its complications. J Hand Surg Am 1988;13:844–9.

29. Bach AW, Almquist EE, Newman DM. Proximal row fusion as a solution for radiocarpal arthritis. J Hand Surg Am 1991;16:424–31.

30. Beyermann K, Prommesberger KJ, Lanz U. Radioscapholunate fusion following comminuted fractures of the distal radius. Eur J Trauma 2000;26:127–43.

31. Nagy L, Buchler U. Long-term results of radioscapholunate fusion following fractures of the distal radius. J Hand Surg Br 1997;22:705–10.

32. O'Bierne J, Boyer MI, Axelrod TS. Wrist arthrodesis using a dynamic compression plate. J Bone Joint Surg Br 1995;77:700–4.

33. Merrell GA, McDermott EM, Weiss AP. Four-corner arthrodesis using a circular plate and distal radius bone grafting: a consecutive case series. J Hand Surg Am 2008;33:635–42.

34. Ashmead D IV, Watson HK, Damon C, et al. Scapholunate advanced collapse wrist salvage. J Hand Surg Am 1994;19:741–50.

35. Bolano LE, Green DP. Wrist arthrodesis in post-traumatic arthritis: a comparison of two methods. J Hand Surg Am 1993;18:700–01.

36. Field J, Herbert TJ, Prosser R. Total wrist fusion. A functional assessment. J Hand Surg Br 1996;21:429–33.

37. Sagerman SD, Palmer AK. Wrist arthrodesis using a dynamic compression plate. J Hand Surg Br 1996;21:437–41.

38. Hartigan BJ, Nagle DJ, Foley MJ. Wrist arthrodesis with excision of the proximal carpal bones using the Ao/ASIF wrist fusion plate and local bone graft. J Hand Surg Br 2001;26:247–51.

39. Meads BM, Scougall PJ, Hargreaves IC. Wrist arthrodesis using a Synthes wrist fusion plate. J Hand Surg Br 2003;28:571–4.

40. Cohen MS, Kozin SH. Degenerative arthritis of the wrist: proximal row carpectomy versus scaphoid excision and four-corner arthrodesis. J Hand Surg Am 2001;26:94–104.

41. Meier R, van Griensven M, Krimmer H. Scaphotrapeziotrapezoid (STT)-arthrodesis in Kienbock's disease. J Hand Surg Br 2004;29:580–4.

42. Watson HK, Weinzweig J, Guidera PM, et al. One thousand intercarpal arthrodeses. J Hand Surg Br 1999;24:307–15.

43. Kleinman WB. Long-term study of chronic scapholunate instability treated by scapho-trapezio-trapezoid arthrodesis. J Hand Surg Am 1989;14:429–45.

44. Borisch N, Haussmann P. Radiolunate arthrodesis in the rheumatoid wrist: a retrospective clinical and radiological longterm follow-up. J Hand Surg Br 2002;27:61–72.

45. Ishikawa H, Hanyu T, Saito H, et al. Limited arthrodesis for the rheumatoid wrist. J Hand Surg Am 1992;17:1103–9.

46. Trumble TE, Easterling KJ, Smith RJ. Ulnocarpal abutment after wrist arthrodesis. J Hand Surg Am 1988;13:11–5.

47. Rogers WD, Watson HK. Radial styloid impingement after triscaphe arthrodesis. J Hand Surg Am 1989;14:297–301.

48. Wollstein R, Watson HK. Scaphotrapeziotrapezoid arthrodesis for arthritis. Hand Clin 2005;21:539–43, vi.

49. Sauerbier M, Kluge S, Bickert B, et al. Subjective and objective outcomes after total wrist arthrodesis in patients with radiocarpal arthrosis or Kienbock's disease. Chir Main 2000;19:223–31.

50. De Smet L, Truyen J. Arthrodesis of the wrist for osteoarthritis: outcome with a minimum follow-up of 4 years. J Hand Surg Br 2003;28:575–7.

51. Tomaino MM, Miller RJ, Burton RI. Outcome assessment following limited wrist fusion: objective wrist scoring versus patient satisfaction. Contemp Orthop 1994;28:403–10.

52. Wyrick JD, Stern PJ, Kiefhaber TR. Motion-preserving procedures in the treatment of scapholunate advanced collapse wrist: proximal row carpectomy versus four-corner arthrodesis. J Hand Surg Am 1995;20:965–70.

Soft Tissue Complications of Distal Radius Fractures

Damien I. Davis, MD[a], Mark Baratz, MD[a,b,c,d,e],*

KEYWORDS

• Distal radius fracture • Soft tissue • Complications • Wrist

Distal radius fractures account for approximately 15% of all fractures in adults. Care of these fractures is associated with a myriad of complications.[1] Complication rates associated with Colles fractures have been reported as high as 31%.[2] There are numerous ways to treat fractures of the distal radius, which include closed reduction and casting, closed reduction and percutaneous pinning, external fixation, and open reduction with internal fixation. Complications associated with each treatment method are unique and being cognizant of them can minimize their eventual occurrence. Complications associated with the soft tissues may be more problematic than the bone injury itself. This review focuses on the soft tissue complications encountered during the management of distal radius fractures, including tendon injury, nerve dysfunction, vascular compromise, skin problems, compartment syndrome, and complex regional pain syndrome.

NEUROVASCULAR DYSFUNCTION

Fractures of the distal radius can affect the median, ulnar, or radial nerves as they cross the wrist, although the median nerve is most frequently affected. Cadaver dissections performed by Vance and Gelberman[3] showed that the distance between the radius and the median nerve decreased as one travels distally down the forearm, from at least 1 cm at the middle of the forearm, to 5 mm at the proximal aspect of the pronator quadratus, to only 3 mm at the level of the wrist. Median nerve injury can occur at the time of injury or during reduction or fixation. Direct injury, such as transection or entrapment of the nerve, is less common than secondary median neuropathy caused by increased carpal tunnel pressure. It is important to differentiate between nerve contusion and compartment syndrome. Compartment syndrome tends to develop slowly with progressively increasing symptoms. Symptoms associated with a median nerve contusion will be present at the time of injury and improve with fracture reduction. Carpal tunnel syndrome can occur acutely, subacutely, or late after distal radius fractures. The incidence of acute transient median nerve compression syndrome sustained after distal radius fracture is estimated to be 4%.[4] The incidence of acute posttraumatic carpal tunnel syndrome requiring urgent decompression is estimated to be between 5.5% and 9% of all distal

[a] Division of Hand & Upper Extremity Surgery, Allegheny General Hospital, Federal North Building, 1307 Federal Street, Second Floor, Pittsburgh, PA 15212, USA
[b] Department of Orthopaedic Surgery, Allegheny General Hospital, 1307 Federal Street, Pittsburgh, PA 15212, USA
[c] Department of Orthopaedic Surgery, Drexel University College of Medicine, 1307 Federal Street, Pittsburgh, PA 19129, USA
[d] Allegheny General Hospital of Upper Extremity Surgery, 1307 Federal Street, Pittsburgh, PA 15212, USA
[e] Allegheny General Hospital Orthopedic Residency & Fellowship Programs, 1307 Federal Street, Pittsburgh, PA 15212, USA
* Corresponding author. Division of Hand & Upper Extremity Surgery, Allegheny General Hospital, Federal North Building, 1307 Federal Street, Second Floor, Pittsburgh, PA 15212.
E-mail address: mbaratz@wpahs.org

Hand Clin 26 (2010) 229–235
doi:10.1016/j.hcl.2009.11.002

radius fractures treated operatively. Dyer and colleagues[5] noted a prevalence of acute carpal tunnel syndrome among patients with a surgically treated fracture of the distal radius of 5.4%. In their analysis, the only significant predictor of acute carpal tunnel syndrome was the amount of fracture translation, specifically in females younger than 48 years.

Acute carpal tunnel syndrome can occur in fractures treated nonoperatively secondary to positioning. The Cotton-Loder position, which entails excessive wrist flexion and ulnar deviation, should be avoided, as a hyperflexed wrist increases the pressure in the carpal tunnel. Gelberman and colleagues[6] showed an average carpal tunnel pressure of 47 mm Hg at 40° flexion compared with 18 mm Hg at neutral flexion. The first step in the initial management of acute carpal tunnel syndrome is placing the wrist in a neutral position with a nonconstrictive dressing. If the median nerve function does not improve, the nerve should be decompressed. Delayed treatment of acute carpal tunnel syndrome can result in permanent median nerve dysfunction. Bauman and colleagues[7] reported complete return of median function in only 1 of 4 operatively treated patients, despite operative intervention within 36 to 96 hours.

The radial nerve can be injured with both nonoperative and operative treatment. A poorly molded splint or cast can result in a radial sensory neuritis secondary to compression at the level of the radial styloid or dorsum of the thumb. The dorsal sensory branch of the radial nerve exits beneath the deep fascia between the brachioradialis and extensor carpi radialis longus, and is prone to injury during percutaneous pining or placement of external fixation pins. Injury to the radial sensory nerve can be avoided by using an open technique, making a small incision, spreading down to bone

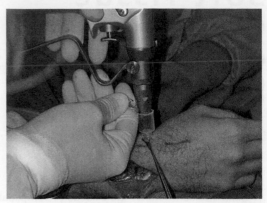

Fig. 2. A drill guide fashioned from a syringe is placed in the small incision over the radial styloid to facilitate K-wire insertion and protect the superficial radial nerve.

and using a drill guide or oscillating drill during pin insertion (**Figs. 1** and **2**).

Injury to the ulnar nerve following a distal radius fracture is rare. The ulnar nerve travels down the forearm under the flexor carpi ulnaris (FCU) and becomes superficial at the level of the FCU tendon; it passes superficial to the transverse carpal ligament, lateral to the pisiform, and then enters the Guyon canal. This anatomic path explains why ulnar nerve dysfunction is less common than that of the median nerve with fractures of the distal radius. At the level of the wrist both the median and ulnar nerves are 3 mm from the radius.[3] However, the median nerve is contained within the carpal tunnel while the ulnar nerve has more available space within the Guyon canal, making it less susceptible to compression. Traumatic ulnar neuropathy tends to be associated with higher energy trauma and more dorsal displacement of the distal radius fragment. Ulnar nerve injuries reported in the literature include severing of the nerve over the sharp edge of the fractured radius, entrapment in the distal radioulnar joint, encasement of the nerve in scar tissue, and displacement of the nerve dorsal to the ulnar styloid.[8–11] Initial treatment of an ulnar nerve palsy following a distal radius fracture is closed reduction of the fracture fragments. If the ulnar nerve function does not improve within 24 to 36 hours, the nerve should be explored with a release of the Guyon canal to minimize the chance of permanent nerve dysfunction.[3]

Complex regional pain syndrome (CRPS) has been associated with distal radius fractures treated both operatively and nonoperatively. CRPS has been associated with overdistraction of the carpus in fractures treated with external fixation. This syndrome is an abnormally intense,

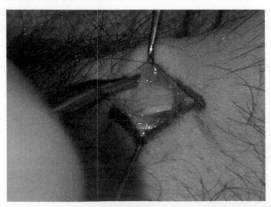

Fig. 1. A small incision over the radial styloid identifies and protects the superficial branch of radial nerve.

prolonged pain response that is disproportionate to the actual tissue damage. The incidence of CRPS after plate fixation of distal radius fractures ranges from 3% to 6%.[12,13] Early intervention should be the focus of treatment. Management includes pain medication, therapy, and sympathetic blocks. The authors' treatment algorithm includes prescribing a Medrol dose pack and a mild analgesic at the first visit. Elavil is added if the patient is experiencing difficulty sleeping. Patients are referred for daily therapy, and instructed to carry something and not isolate the affected hand. Then they are rechecked in 48 hours if they are not sleeping or in 1 week if their sleep is not disturbed. If the pain is improved and the patient feels as if he or she is getting better, therapy is continued. If the pain is refractory, the patient is referred for a sympathetic stellate ganglion block. A recent study by Zollinger and colleagues[14] showed a decreased rate of CRPS in wrist fracture patients treated with vitamin C for 50 days after injury.

Acute vascular injuries associated with fractures of the distal radius are exceedingly rare. Case reports have described entrapment of the ulnar artery preventing fracture reduction, dorsal displacement of the ulnar artery around the ulnar styloid, and radial artery pseudoaneurysm with subsequent microembolism to the thumb.[11,15,16]

SKIN

A large percentage of fractures of the distal radius are fragility fractures, occurring in an older patient population. This population, along with patients with inflammatory arthropathy or taking systemic corticosteroids, possess fragile skin and are more vulnerable to complications stemming from the fracture itself or the subsequent treatment. Tearing of the skin may occur during manual reduction of the fracture. Performing the closed reduction under regional or general anesthesia improves muscle relaxation and enables a gentler reduction maneuver, decreasing the potential for skin tearing. The majority of skin complications associated with distal radius fractures arises from problems secondary to splint or cast application. Complications due to casting include stiffness, pressure sores, and compartment syndrome. As a general rule, sugar tong splints should be applied in the acute setting of a distal radius fracture, followed by delayed casting once the potential for further swelling is minimal.

Infection is a known complication of any surgical procedure. Whereas it is rarely reported with plate fixation, it is more prevalent with percutaneous pinning and external fixation. Hargreaves and colleagues[17] reported superficial pin site infection rates of 34% when the Kirschner wires were left out of the skin, and 7% when the wires were buried. Pin site infections ranging from 21% to 37% have been reported with external fixators.[18,19] Ahlborg and colleagues[19] recommend removing percutaneous Kirschner wires by 8 weeks.

COMPARTMENT SYNDROME

Compartment syndrome is a rare complication following fracture of the distal end of the radius, with a prevalence of less than 1%.[2] Potential sites of compartment syndrome include the hand and forearm. There are ten separate osteofascial compartments of the hand: 4 dorsal interossei, 3 volar interossei, the adductor pollicus, and the thenar and hypothenar muscle groups. Traditional anatomic texts describe the forearm as containing 3 distinct compartments: volar, dorsal, and mobile wad. The volar compartment has been further subdivided into superficial and deep compartments. More recently, a third anatomically distinct volar compartment has been described, the pronator quadratus compartment.[20] Compartment syndrome can theoretically occur in any of the aforementioned compartments, but it is seen most frequently in the volar compartment of the forearm. Compartment syndrome has been reported following closed reduction and immobilization, open reduction and internal fixation, and external fixation. Compartment syndrome is most commonly seen, prior to treatment, as a result of high energy trauma. Acute compartment of dorsal and volar compartments has been reported following a low energy fall.[21]

Diagnosis of compartment syndrome is primarily based on clinical findings. Intracompartmental pressure measurements are a useful confirmatory test, but should not substitute for a thorough physical examination. Physical examination findings include tense compartments, pain out of proportion to the injury, and pain with passive stretch of the involved compartment. In cases of suspected compartment syndrome, patients should be monitored closely with attention to the neurovascular examination and pain medication requirements. Compartment syndrome associated with a distal radius fracture has been reported to occur from 12 to 54 hours after the initial injury.[22,23] Regional anesthesia may mask the symptoms of compartment syndrome and this must be considered when monitoring patients postoperatively.

Initial treatment of compartment syndrome should be to relieve circumferential pressure by splitting the cast or loosening the splint. Plaster cast cutting and spreading can reduce pressures by 40% to 60%. Release of the padding underneath may reduce the pressure an additional 10% to 20%.[24,25] Operative fasciotomy is required if symptomatic improvement after the release of casts and constrictive bandages does not occur. The incision for the volar compartment fasciotomy begins proximally at the antecubital fossa to release the lacertus fibrosus, and extends distally down the forearm in a curvilinear manner to terminate in the palm to facilitate the release of the carpal tunnel. A volar forearm fasciotomy will often reduce pressures in the dorsal compartments. However, if dorsal compartment pressures remain elevated, a dorsal, linear, longitudinal forearm incision is made between the mobile extensor wad and the extensor digitorum communis muscle bellies to release both compartments. Delayed diagnosis or treatment of forearm compartment syndrome can have catastrophic consequences, resulting in Volkmann ischemic contracture and muscle loss with significant functional compromise.

TENDON INJURY

Tendon injury following a distal radius fracture is a rare complication. However, recently the frequency of tendon injury has increased as volar locking plates have become more popular. Injuries to flexor and extensor tendons can range from adhesion formation to simple irritation to frank rupture. Tendon complications have been reported in both conservatively treated and operatively treated fractures. Rupture of the extensor pollicus longus (EPL) during closed treatment of a nondisplaced distal radius fracture was first described by Duplay in 1876. The reported incidence of this complication is 0.07% to 0.88%.[26,27] The interval between fracture and tendon rupture ranges from days to years, but usually occurs within 8 weeks from the initial injury. The 2 proposed etiologies of this rupture are a mechanical theory and a vascular theory. Pundits of the mechanical theory have suggested that rupture results from a prominent edge of the dorsal cortex protruding into the third extensor compartment. Tendon injury according to the vascular theory is thought to occur in a vascular watershed area of the EPL tendon subjected to high-stress decreased third extensor compartment perfusion secondary to increased pressure from fracture callus and hematoma, or systemic factors such as systemic corticosteroid use that may alter blood flow to the tendon.[28]

Engkvist and Lundborg[28] described the vascularity of the EPL tendon as almost entirely intrinsic, with 2 longitudinal vessels running within the tendon from both its proximal and distal aspects. As these 2 systems converge near the Lister tubercle, there is an area of the tendon approximately 0.5 cm length without any vessels. Engkvist and Lundborg determined that this relatively avascular segment corresponds to the level of the rupture of the tendon, and also postulated that the anatomic course of the EPL tendon could be partially responsible for the susceptibility to injury. As the EPL tendon passes dorsally in the third extensor compartment, it takes a sharp turn around the ulnar aspect of the Lister tubercle. This angular course is subject to bending and torsional forces which could, in a tendon with compromised vascularity, contribute to its rupture.

Rupture of extensor tendons is also possible during or after treating a distal radius fracture with a volar plate. Sources of injury include drill-bit penetration and prominent dorsal screw tips (**Fig. 3**). The problem with prominent dorsal screw tips stems from 2 characteristics of distal radius fractures. First, it is difficult to determine screw length with a depth gauge when the dorsal cortex is comminuted. Second, screws penetrating the dorsal cortex that are at the same level as the Lister tubercle can appear contained within the bone on a lateral projection. Benson and colleagues[29] performed a retrospective review to evaluate techniques to minimize damage to the EPL tendon during volar plating of the distal radius. These investigators determined that screws 2 mm longer than the measured depth did not appear prominent on lateral images. The screw lengths needed to be at least 4 mm longer than the measured depth to observe penetration of the dorsal cortex. Benson and colleagues[29] suggested using shorter screws in the holes directed

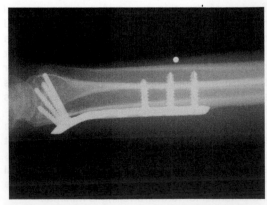

Fig. 3. Prominent dorsal screw tips of the proximal 2 shaft screws. These screws caused a tendonitis of the second extensor compartment, mimicking an overuse-type intersection syndrome.

toward the third extensor compartment, and proposed making a small incision just ulnar to the Lister tubercle to visually inspect the third compartment for prominent hardware after plate application in patients with dorsal comminution (**Fig. 4**). Complete rupture of any tendon may be preceded by tenderness or swelling over the tendon. If EPL tendonitis is suspected, exploration and decompression, or hardware removal if prominent, may prevent rupture. If rupture does occur, primary repair is not possible given the frayed tendon ends. Thumb extension can be restored by transferring the extensor indicis proprius tendon to the EPL tendon or reconstructing the tendon with an intercalary tendon graft.

EPL ruptures are the most frequently reported extensor tendon complications, but extensor digitorum communis tendon ruptures, intersection syndrome, and extensor tenosynovitis associated with fractures of the distal radius have all been described. In addition, extensor tendon entrapment (**Fig. 5**) can also occur, specifically with injury to the distal radioulnar joint (DRUJ). The extensor carpi ulnaris and extensor digiti minimi have both been described as becoming interposed in the DRUJ. Entrapment of an extensor tendon in the DRUJ may be radiographically apparent as a widened DRUJ or clinically as a vacant extensor carpi ulnaris (ECU) sulcus over the distal ulna. This vacant ECU sulcus is referred to as the "empty sulcus sign."[30] The DRUJ remains irreducible, despite reduction and fixation of the radius fracture. Definitive fixation requires reduction of the DRUJ and repair of the extensor carpi ulnaris tendon sheath to optimize stability.

Flexor tendon injury following distal radius fracture is less common than extensor tendon injury. Nonetheless, flexor carpi radialis, flexor pollicus longus, flexor digitorum superficialis, and flexor digitorum profundus tendon ruptures have been

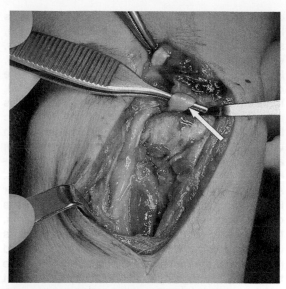

Fig. 5. The arrow indicates the extensor tendon entrapped within the fracture site. (*Courtesy of* Terry Light, MD, Maywood, IL.)

reported as both acute and delayed complications of distal radius fractures.[31] The anatomy is thought to be partly responsible for the relative paucity of flexor tendon injuries compared with those of the extensor tendons. Flexor tendons are not as tightly enclosed over the distal aspect of the radius, and the pronator quadratus may serve to protect the flexor tendons from injury secondary to sharp bone edges. Distal to the edge of the pronator quadratus and proximal to the volar radiocarpal ligaments lies a transverse ridge known as the watershed line. The watershed line is within 2 mm from the articular surface on the ulnar aspect of the radius and 10 to 15 mm from the radial articular surface. The clinical significance of this area is that hardware placed distal to the watershed line can abut the flexor tendons and can increase the risk of tendonitis or rupture. In a study by Arora and colleagues[4] implants were placed over or distal to the watershed line in 11 patients and all developed tendon problems, either synovitis or rupture. These investigators recommended early removal of the hardware if the distal aspect of the plate is prominent or becomes prominent due to collapse of the fracture. Arora and colleagues also suggested early plate removal in patients who were on a long-standing regimen of steroids.[32–35]

LIGAMENT DYSFUNCTION

Chronic DRUJ instability is a known complication after distal radius fractures, particularly in those

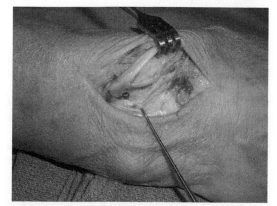

Fig. 4. The dorsal incision shows the prominent screw tip within the third extensor compartment.

cases where the radius has malunited. There is little inherent bony stability to the DRUJ. Hence, soft tissues such as the pronator quadratus, extensor carpi ulnaris, interosseous membrane, DRUJ capsule, and triangular fibrocartilage comprise the majority of support for the DRUJ. Inadequate healing of the soft tissue structures after a distal radius fracture may result in chronic DRUJ instability. Patients may present with ulnar-sided wrist pain, loss of forearm rotation, and decreased grip strength. Nonsurgical treatment of chronic DRUJ instability is usually futile. A trial of immobilization in a sugar tong splint or long arm cast can be attempted for milder cases of instability, especially in lower demand patients. If nonoperative treatment is unsuccessful, it is useful to determine whether there is an associated malunion of the distal radius which can contribute to DRUJ incongruity and instability. In recent injuries, mild instability may be correctable with triangular fibrocartilage complex (TFCC) repair alone. Gross instability suggests a more extensive injury to the capsule surrounding the DRUJ and the interosseous membrane. In this scenario, TFCC repair may need to be augmented with repair of the capsule and, if necessary, pinning the radius to the ulna proximal to the DRUJ for 4 weeks. Chronic cases of mild instability can be managed with TFCC repair. Mild chronic instability with no TFCC tear can be managed with an ulnar shortening osteotomy. In chronic injuries with gross instability, it has been the authors' experience that either TFCC repair or ulnar shortening osteotomy alone is ineffective. The authors manage gross, chronic DRUJ instability with ligament reconstruction combined with a sigmoid notchplasty if the notch appears hypoplastic on computed tomography.

Malunited fractures that include significant degrees of shortening or angulation are treated with corrective osteotomy. After the osteotomy is fixed with a plate, stability of the DRUJ is reassessed. The aforementioned algorithm applies to the corrected malunion with persistent instability of the DRUJ.

A contraindication to soft tissue reconstruction is an arthritic sigmoid notch. In these instances, salvage procedure including distal ulnar resection, the Sauve-Kapandji procedure or arthroplasty of the DRUJ, may be performed with great care to optimize soft tissue stability.[36]

SUMMARY

Although a fracture of the distal radius is primarily thought of as bone problem, it is important to be cognizant of the potential soft tissue complications that are associated with this injury to optimize outcomes. A thorough physical examination is necessary on initial evaluation and during follow-up to address any tendon injury, nerve dysfunction, vascular compromise, skin problem, compartment syndrome, CRPS, or ligament dysfunction that may arise.

ACKNOWLEDGMENTS

The authors would like to acknowledge Anne Morgan Selleck for her help and contributions in preparation of this article.

REFERENCES

1. Lofthus CM, Frihagen F, Meyer HE, et al. Epidemiology of distal forearm fractures in Oslo, Norway. Osteoporos Int 2008;19:781–6.
2. Cooney WP III, Dobyns JH, Linschied RL. Complications of Colles' fractures. J Bone Joint Surg Am 1980;62:613–9.
3. Vance RM, Gelberman RH. Acute ulnar neuropathy with fractures at the wrist. J Bone Joint Surg Am 1978;60:962–5.
4. Arora R, Lutz M, Hennerbichler A, et al. Complications following internal fixation of unstable distal radius fracture with a palmar locking-plate. J Orthop Trauma 2007;21(5):316–22.
5. Dyer G, Lozano-Calderon S, Gannon C, et al. Predictors of acute carpal tunnel syndrome associated with fractures of the distal radius. J Hand Surg 2008;33(8):1309–13.
6. Gelberman RH, Szabo RM, Mortensen WW. Carpal tunnel pressures and wrist position in patients with Colles' fractures. J Trauma 1984;24(8):747–9.
7. Bauman TD, Gelberman RH, Mubarak SJ, et al. The acute carpal tunnel syndrome. Clin Orthop Relat Res 1981;156:151–6.
8. Pazart F, Stindel E, Le Nen D. Fracture of the distal part of the radius associated with severed ulnar nerve. Chir Main 1999;18:197–201.
9. Clarke AC, Spencer RF. Ulnar nerve palsy following fractures of the distal radius: clinical and anatomical studies. J Hand Surg Br 1991;16:438–40.
10. Poppi M, Padovani R, Martinelli P, et al. Fracture of the distal radius with ulnar nerve palsy. J Trauma 1978;18:278–9.
11. Sohal JK, Chia B, Catalano LW. Dorsal displacement of the ulnar nerve after a displaced distal radius fracture: case report. J Hand Surg Am 2009;34:432–5.
12. Drobetz H, Kutscha-Lissberg E. Osteosynthesis of distal radius fractures with a volar locking screw plate system. Int Orthop 2003;27:1–6.

13. Kamano M, Koshimune M, Toyama M, et al. Palmar plating system for Colles' fractures—a preliminary report. J Hand Surg 2005;30:750–5.

14. Zollinger PE, Tuinebreijer WE, Breederveld RS, et al. Can vitamin C prevent complex regional pain syndrome in patients with wrist fractures? A randomized, controlled multicenter dose-response study. J Bone Joint Surg 2007;89:1424–31.

15. Fernandez DL. Irreducible radiocarpal fracture-dislocation and radioulnar dissociation with entrapment of the ulnar nerve, artery, and flexor profundus II-V—a case report. J Hand Surg Am 1981;6:456–61.

16. Dao KD, Venn-Watson E, Shin AY. Radial artery pseudoaneurysm complication from use of AO/ASIF volar distal radius plate: a case report. J Hand Surg Am 2001;26:448–53.

17. Hargreaves DG, Drew SJ, Eckersley R. Kirschner wire pin tract infection rates: a randomized controlled trial between percutaneous and buried wires. J Hand Surg Br 2004;29(4):374–6.

18. Anderson JT, Lucas GL, Buhr BR. Complications of treating distal radius fractures with external fixation: a community experience. Iowa Orthop J 2004;24:53–9.

19. Ahlborg HG, Josefsson PO. Pin-tract complications in external fixation of fractures of the distal radius. Acta Orthop Scand 1999;70(2):116–8.

20. Sotereanos DG, McCarthy DM, Towers JD, et al. The pronator quadratus: a distinct forearm space? J Hand Surg Am 1995;20:496–9.

21. Kupersmith LM, Weinfeld SB. Acute volar and dorsal compartment syndrome after a distal radius fracture: a case report. J Orthop Trauma 2003;17:382–6.

22. Simpson NS, Jupiter JB. Delayed onset of forearm compartment syndrome: a complication of distal radius fracture in young adults. J Orthop Trauma 1995;9(5):411–8.

23. Stockley I, Harvey IA, Getty CJ. Acute volar compartment syndrome of the forearm secondary to fractures of the distal radius. Injury 1988;19(2):101–4.

24. Garfin SR, Mubarak SJ, Evans KL, et al. Quantification of intracompartmental pressure and volume under plaster casts. J Bone Joint Surg Am 1981; 63:449–53.

25. Halanski M, Noonan KJ. Cast and splint immobilization: complications. J Am Acad Orthop Surg 2008; 16:30–40.

26. Heidemann J, Gausepohl T, Pennig D. Narrowing of the third extensor tendon compartment in minimal displaced distal radius fractures with impending rupture of the EPL tendon. Handchir Mikrochir Plast Chir 2002;34:324–7 [in German].

27. Hove LM. Delayed rupture of the thumb extensor tendon: a 5 year study of 1 consecutive cases. Acta Orthop Scand 1994;65:199–203.

28. Engkvist O, Lundborg G. Rupture of the extensor pollicus longus tendon after fracture of the lower end of the radius: a clinical and microangiographic study. Hand 1979;11:76–86.

29. Benson EC, DeCarvalho A, Mikola EA, et al. Two potential causes of EPL rupture after distal radius volar plate fixation. Clin Orthop Relat Res 2006; 451:218–22.

30. Paley D, McMurtry RY, Murray JF. Dorsal dislocation of the ulnar styloid and extensor carpi ulnaris tendon into the distal radioulnar joint: the empty sulcus sign. J Hand Surg Am 1987;12:1029–32.

31. DiMatteo L, wolf JM. Flexor carpi radialis tendon rupture as a complication of a closed distal radius fracture: a case report. J Hand Surg Am 2007; 32(6):818–20.

32. Bell JS, Wollstein R, Cintron ND. Rupture of the flexor pollicis longus tendon: a complication of volar plating of the distal radius. J Bone Joint Surg Br 1998;80:225–6.

33. Koo SC, Ho ST. Delayed rupture of flexor pollicis longus tendon after volar plating of the distal radius. Hand Surg 2006;11:67–70.

34. Berglund LM, Messer TM. Complications of volar plate fixation for managing distal radius fractures. J Am Acad Orthop Surg 2009;17(6):369–77.

35. Kozin SH, Wood MB. Early soft tissue complications after fractures of the distal part of the radius. J Bone Joint Surg Am 1993;75:144–53.

36. Adams BD, Lawler E. Chronic instability of the distal radioulnar joint. J Am Acad Orthop Surg 2007;15: 571–5.

Complications Associated with Distraction Plate Fixation of Wrist Fractures

Douglas P. Hanel, MD[a],*, Scott David Ruhlman, MD[a],
Leo I. Katolik, MD[b], Christopher H. Allan, MD[a]

KEYWORDS

- Distal radius • Bridge plate • Distraction plate
- Complications • Fracture • Comminuted • External fixation

With the advent of volar plate and fragment-specific fixation of wrist fractures, the role of joint-spanning fixation has become increasingly limited. Despite its waning popularity, spanning fixation in the form of external fixation and internal plates has proven to be an effective method for treating fractures of the distal radius in the setting of severely comminuted fractures, polytraumatized patients and, at times, the elderly.[1–4] By "off-loading" the radiocarpal joint, distraction-fixation allows weight bearing through the affected limb, without compromising the radius fracture reduction. This procedure effectively minimizes the medical complications of immobility and allows for earlier independence in transfers.

Despite results comparable to other fixation techniques, enthusiasm for external fixation is tempered by pin tract complications, occurring in 10% to 54% of cases, and the myriad of complications associated with the treatment of wrist fractures, including finger and wrist joint stiffness, metacarpal fractures, nonunions, nerve injuries, dystrophic pain, and implant failure.[2–21]

By using an internal plate that spans the radiocarpal joint, most implant-related complications can be circumvented. In 2 recent studies, an internal plate affixed to the radial shaft proximally and the second or third metacarpal distally

effectively recapitulated the benefits of external fixation and served as an adjunct to internal fixation in the clinical setting of polytrauma and combined intra-articular metadiaphyseal injuries.[22–24] In these studies the internal plate was referred to as a bridge plate or distraction plate. In this article this technique is referred to as distraction plating. Distraction plating was associated with minimal complications in these clinical studies, and was proven to have superior fixation properties when compared with external fixation in later biomechanical studies.[25]

As enthusiastic as these published studies are, they reflect the clinical acumen of the senior investigators in small cohort studies. The authors wondered if this success and, more importantly, these minimal complications could be reflected in the application of these techniques by multiple surgeons at the authors' level I trauma center. The following study attempts to answer these questions.

MATERIALS AND METHODS

After obtaining approval from the Institutional Review Board, the authors retrospectively reviewed all patients undergoing bridge distraction plate fixation of distal radius fractures by 3

---

[a] Department of Orthopaedics and Sports Medicine, University of Washington, PO Box 359798, 325 Ninth Avenue, Seattle, WA 98102, USA
[b] Department of Orthopaedic Surgery, Thomas Jefferson University School of Medicine, Philadelphia, PA, USA
* Corresponding author.
E-mail address: dhanel@uw.edu

Hand Clin 26 (2010) 237–243
doi:10.1016/j.hcl.2010.01.001
0749-0712/10/$ – see front matter © 2010 Elsevier Inc. All rights reserved.

surgeons in a single level I trauma center. The patients were selected and reviewed between June 2001 and July 2007; charts and radiographs were reviewed.

Indications for distraction plating included one or all of the following scenarios: (1) unstable fractures of the distal radius, associated with polytrauma, in patients who would benefit from using the upper extremities to assist with weight bearing, (2) bilateral wrist fractures that were severely comminuted and extended into the radial diaphysis, and (3) combined-complex injuries requiring extensive soft tissue and bony reconstruction. A typical clinical example is shown in **Fig. 1**.

Plates were removed when the fractures healed, and all patients in the study were followed at least until that time. Most patients were followed well beyond fracture healing, reflecting the typical course for recovery of motion, strength, and endurance that occurs after skeletal healing. Patients were excluded from the study if they did not have documented removal of the distraction plate.

Technique

All fractures were treated with dorsally placed distraction plates using a previously described technique.[22] While under general or regional anesthesia, the fracture is grossly realigned with 4.5 kg of longitudinal traction. This realignment is followed by a reduction technique described by John Agee MD: longitudinal traction restores length, palmar translation of the hand relative to the forearm restores palmar tilt, and pronation of the hand relative to the radius corrects the radiocarpal supination deformity.[26] In the more severely comminuted fractures, the latter 2 maneuvers served to confirm the global instability of the fracture, resulting in unabated palmar translation of the hand relative to the forearm. In the less severe cases, the articular alignment is restored and secured with K-wires passed percutaneously. If articular fragments cannot be reduced while closed then the fracture site is opened, and the articular fracture reduced and secured with

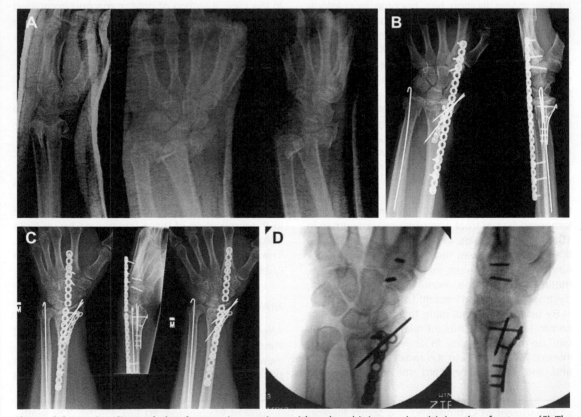

Fig. 1. (*A*) Distal radius and ulna fracture in a patient with a closed injury and multiple other fractures. (*B*) The fracture is reduced and secured with a volar buttress plate. The ulna is secured with an intermedullary fixation wire. (*C*) Six weeks after injury the patient returned to heavy labor and ranching. Despite notification, he refused to return for plate removal. Twenty months after injury he returned for evaluation of swelling on the dorsum of the hand. (*D*) The distraction plate and readily accessible K-wires and screws were removed. At 6 years post injury he reports minimal pain, and continues all work activities and avocations.

K-wires, screws or plates, and screws. The distraction plate is then applied.

A 4-cm incision is made over the second or third metacarpal and the distraction plate is slid underneath the second or fourth extensor compartment, and aligned to the radial diaphysis proximally. The choice of second versus fourth compartment depends on the fracture characteristics and the surgeon's preference. A proximal incision, 4 cm long, is made along the radial diaphysis in line with the proximal holes of the distraction plate. The plate position is confirmed with image intensification. The plate is first lagged down to the metacarpal distally and radius proximally using nonlocking cortical screws. If locking screws are available, they are incorporated into the plate at this time. The distal radioulnar joint is then addressed, and reconstructed when necessary then splinted in forearm supination for the first 2 weeks after surgery. K-wires are removed 6 weeks postoperatively, and the distraction plate is removed after radiographic union, usually within 3 to 4 months of injury. Patients are allowed to bear weight through the forearm and flexed elbow when other injuries allow and when platform crutches can be used to assist with ambulation. After 3 weeks, when elbow and forearm motion is no longer restricted by splints, the platform is removed and weight bearing by using the grip handles of the crutch is allowed.

RESULTS

During the study period, there were 912 consecutive patients who underwent operative treatment of distal radius fractures. Of these, 140 patients (15%) with 144 fractures were treated with a dorsally placed distraction plate. A Synthes 2.4-mm titanium "mandibular" plate (Synthes Inc, West Chester, PA, USA) was used in the first 59 fractures, whereas a custom 2.7-mm stainless steel locking plate was used in the remaining fractures.

The average age at the time of injury was 48.5 years (range, 19–95 years) with 86 (66.2%) fractures occurring in male patients and 44 (33.8%) fractures in female patients. The mechanism of injury was a fall from height in 89 (68%), motor vehicle accident in 22 (17.1%), motorcycle crash in 9 (7.1%), pedestrian versus vehicle in 7 (5.4%), plane crash in 2 (1.6%), and direct blow to the arm in 1 (0.8%).

Additional fixation was used in 74 cases (57%). K-wires alone were used in 62 (48%) cases, K-wires and a volar plate in 7 (9.5%), K-wires with supplemental cancellous allograft in 2 (1.5%), and K-wires and fragmentary screw fixation in 2 (1.5%). Supplemental cancellous allograft alone was used in 1 (0.8%) case.

There were 13 patients with open fractures, all of whom were treated on the day of injury, and the wound closed within 3 days of definitive fixation. Two patients who presented with forearm compartmental syndromes underwent forearm and hand fasciotomies, and fracture fixation. Split-thickness skin grafts were used to close these wounds within 3 days after fixation. No patient required distant flap coverage.

Eighty-nine patients had associated acute injuries to other extremities or organ systems that required treatment. Of these, 17 patients had abdominal injuries, 15 had chest injuries, 25 had head injuries, and 13 had a combination of head, chest, and abdominal injuries; 54 patients had weight-bearing restrictions resulting from pelvis or lower extremity injuries, and 46 patients had at least one other operative procedure unrelated to distal radius fractures.

Of these 144 patients, 10 were excluded from review due to lack of follow-up. These included 2 patients who died of the sequelae of polytrauma, 1 who refused to have his plate removed, and 7 who left the region. Of these 7 patients, 4 provided erroneous information and could not be contacted, and the remaining 3 patients had their plate removed locally and refused to participate in final evaluation. The remaining 130 patients with fractures were followed until the completion of the study.

The average time from plate insertion to plate removal was 136 days (range, 49–809 days), for an average of 43 weeks; this was an average of 24 weeks after plate removal.

Complications were divided into 2 groups, major and minor. Major complications are defined as those requiring additional unanticipated operative intervention. Minor complications are defined as those that did not require additional operative procedures. There were a total of 16 (12.3%) complications in 15 patients with 16 fractures, 7 (5.3%) minor and 9 (6.9%) major (**Tables 1** and **2**).

Minor Complications

Hardware failure complicated 5 fractures. In 3 fractures, the plate fractured at the radiocarpal articulation through an empty screw hole. This problem occurred an average of 10 months after plate application (range, 5–20 months) and in each case the fracture had healed before plate failure (see **Fig. 1**). Two patients sustained metacarpal fractures through distal fixation screw holes, prior to wrist fracture healing and plate removal; one, presumably, due to voluntary return

Table 1
Major and minor complications

Minor Complications	
Wound healing	2
Hardware failure without loss of reduction	5
Total	7
Major Complications	
Malunion	2
Nonunion requiring surgery	2
Wound complications, unplanned surgery	1
Deep infection	2
Extensor tendon adhesions, tenolysis	2
EPL rupture requiring EIP transfer	1
Total	10

Abbreviations: EIP, extensor indicis proprius; EPL, extensor pollicis longus.

to heavy labor and the other due to severe osteoporosis. Both of these fractures were treated closed and were healed when the plate was removed. No plate or screw failure was associated with tendon rupture.

Major Complications

Two cases of deep infection required early hardware removal, 3 to 4 weeks after placement. The infections resolved with multiple debridements and antibiotics. Both cases were closed fractures in polytraumatized patients. Both fractures maintained reduction and healed. There were 2 cases of symptomatic malunion and 2 cases of nonunion that required additional surgeries. Symptomatic malunions included 1 case of a distal radioulnar joint step-off and 1 case of a 7-mm shortened but healed distal radius. The first patient refused further treatment and the other was treated with a distal ulna resection interposition arthroplasty. One of the patients with delayed unions was treated with an iliac crest autograft, which healed, and then had the distraction plate removed. The other case had the distraction plate removed and a volar plate applied. No bone graft was used and this fracture united.

One case of delayed extensor pollicis longus rupture was thought to result from fracture callous, and was treated with excision of the offending bone and an extensor indicis proprius tendon transfer. Two cases with limited metacarpal phalangeal joint motion required extensive tenolysis at the time of plate removal. Joint motion returned to normal.

Patients whose plates were left in place for longer than 16 weeks had an overall complication rate of 20.8%, compared with an overall complication rate of 8.5% in those whose plates could be removed before 16 weeks. This difference, although remarkable on first impression, is not statistically significant ($P = .138$).

The occurrence of complications was evenly distributed throughout the series; 8 complications occurred in the first 65 fractures and 9 complications occurred in the next 65 fractures.

There were no pathologic fractures of the radial or metacarpal shafts after hardware removal.

DISCUSSION

There is currently no evidence to suggest the superiority of a single technique for the treatment of distal radius fractures, and this article does not seek to suggest the superiority of dorsal bridge plate fixation over other techniques. In the authors' institution, many fixation techniques are used and each is carefully matched to the personality of the fracture type, the general injury pattern, and the patients' overall health and rehabilitative imperatives. The authors believe that the rote application of one implant or technique is misguiding. However, in those circumstances in which surgeons consider external fixation, the authors advocate dorsal bridge plate fixation instead.

In the authors' institution distraction plate fixation is used for 2 specific groups of wrist injuries, in those with highly comminuted metadiaphyseal fractures and in those whose polytrauma requires weight bearing with a limb that also has a wrist fracture. Recent modification in the available diaphyseal lengths of implants designed for the volar wrist may supplant the need for distraction plating in the first group, but not in the second. No intra-articular fracture construct that does not span the radiocarpal joint can withstand the rigors of weight bearing. The spanning plate distracts the articulation between the radius and the carpus and prevents displacement of articular fractures and subsidence, or hardware failure.

The most frequently reported adjunct to the treatment of wrist fractures in the setting of multiple traumas is external fixation. Despite excellent results, even when compared with all the other forms of distal radius treatment, external fixation has been plagued with the highest complication rates reported in the management of distal radius fractures.[3–6] The most commonly reported complication is pin tract infections. A typical example is the 1986 report of Weber and Szabo,[27] who showed a major complication rate of 62% and called for consideration of alternative treatment methods. Other equally disappointing rates of pin tract complications are included in the studies by

Table 2
Details of patients' complications

Age/Sex	Mechanism	Open	Complication	Treatment
Minor Complications				
29 M	MCC	No	Wound dehiscence	Dressing changes
80 F	6-ft fall	No	Distal wound breakdown	Dressing changes
53 M	MCC	No	Distal screw failure, fx healed	Plate removed
58 F	6-ft fall	No	Distal fixation failure, fx healed	Plate removed
57 M	20-ft fall	Yes	Broken plate and screws, 20 mo post fixation	Plate removed
85 F	6-ft fall	No	Bilateral fx plate break after fx healed	Plate removed
85 F	6-ft fall	No	Same patient as above	
Major Complications				
37 M	10-ft fall	No	Deep infection	Plate removed IV antibiotics
27 M	25-ft fall	Yes	Late deep infection, fx healed	Plate removed oral antibiotics
55 M	8-ft fall	Yes	Malunion healed, 7 mm short	Refused revision
32 M	20-ft fall	No	Painful DRUJ malunion	Distal ulna resection
40 M	MCC	Yes	Nonunion	Autograft graft, then plate removal
44 M	10-ft fall	Yes	Radius metaphyseal nonunion	Change to volar plate
22 M	30-ft fall	Yes	Unstable scar, 1 year post	Resection
62 M	MCC	No	EPL adhesions	Plate removal and tenolysis
48 M	30-ft fall	No	Extensor adhesions	Plate removal and tenolysis

Abbreviations: DRUJ, distal radioulnar joint; fx, fracture; MCC, motorcycle car collision.

Sanders and colleagues,[19] 14 of 35 (40%); Hutchinson and colleagues,[9] 26 of 50 (52%); and Anderson and colleagues,[11] 16 of 24 (67%). Even in less dramatic series the pin tract complications alone are reported to be 11%.[4,13,15]

In 2008, Handoll and Madhok[3] reviewed the Cochrane Database and identified 8 prospective randomized controlled studies in which external fixator complications of distal radius fixation were reported. In 352 patients over the 8 studies, 87 (25%) had significant pin tract complications.

Although pin tract complications might be considered minor, it is these complications that most often limit the period of time for which an external fixator can remain in place, usually 5 to 7 weeks. With distraction plate fixation, implant removal is not considered until fracture consolidation has been confirmed. The plate is then removed at the convenience of the patient and not because of the urgency of complications such as pin tract infections. This is reflected in the study of Ruch and colleagues,[23,24] who reported consolidation occurring at an average of 110 days after fixation and distraction plate removal at an average of 14 days later.

In this study the complications of a cohort of patients treated by board certified surgeons, who were familiar with wrist fracture fixation but had a variable level of familiarity using distraction plating techniques, are critically reviewed. The authors believe that this study demonstrates an acceptable complication rate. There were 2 delayed unions in this series and each reflected the severity of the original injury more than the fixation technique. Each delayed union responded to routine intervention with bone grafts or augmented fracture stabilization. Similarly, the 2 malunions presented with the fracture reflect the severity of the injury, an unreconstructable distal radioulnar joint in 1 case and a severely comminuted radial metaphysis in the other. The infection rate in 2 of the 130 fractures is certainly superior to the infection rate associated with external fixation discussed earlier. The fixation failure in these cases is bothersome. In each case, fixation plates and screws failed after fracture healing, but preceded fracture plate removal. This situation reflects the increased activity that comes with the comfort of a healed fracture and increased use. In the case of plate failure, the 2.7-mm implant, in which empty screw holes in the plate were adjacent to the radiocarpal joint, broke. This break can be avoided by using a larger implant, a 3.5-mm plate, or by manufacturing an implant that does not have empty screw holes in the midportion of the implant. Such an implant is presently only available through custom manufacturing. The authors also found that 2.4-mm screws, whether titanium or stainless steel, will break at the interface between the plate and the bone that they are engaging. This problem is avoided by using plate fixation screws no smaller than 2.7 mm. Finally, the number of complications related to the timing of plate removal was elevated in those patients who had their plates removed later than 16 weeks. Just like all of the complications discussed earlier, this reflects severity of injury leading to delayed fracture healing and in the case of an 85-year-old woman with bilateral fractures, a desire to avoid further surgery (**Fig. 2**). The authors recommend that distraction plates can be removed within weeks of radiographic evidence of healing, and sooner if there is evidence of plate breakage. The location of a broken plate at the radiocarpal articulation portends the disastrous potential of tendon rupture.

The value of this study is limited by 2 potential reporting biases. The first is the lack of follow-up beyond 43 weeks. The authors think that most procedure-related complications should be seen by 43 weeks, on average 24 weeks after plate

removal. The second potential bias is that the complications reviewed and presented are the results of cases performed by the same surgeons reporting them. An attempt was made to minimize this bias by recruiting a senior orthopedic resident to review all the cases and confirm the complication with senior surgeons not associated with the case(s).

In summary, this article identifies that dorsally placed distraction plates can be used effectively and safely, with a major complication rate of 8.5% and a minor complication rate of 4.6%. The major disadvantage to distraction plating is the need for plate removal as a second procedure.

REFERENCES

1. Edwards GS Jr. Intra-articular fractures of the distal part of the radius treated with the small AO external fixator. J Bone Joint Surg Am 1991;73(8):1241–50.
2. Graff S, Jupiter J. Fracture of the distal radius: classification of treatment and indications for external fixation. Injury 1994;25(Suppl 4):S-D14–25.
3. Handoll HH, Madhok R. Surgical interventions for treating distal radial fractures in adults. Cochrane Database Syst Rev 2001;(3):CD003209.
4. Egol K, Walsh M, Tejwani N, et al. Bridging external fixation and supplementary Kirschner-wire fixation versus volar locked plating for unstable fractures of the distal radius: a randomised, prospective trial. J Bone Joint Surg Br 2008;90(9):1214–21.
5. Grewal R, Perey B, Wilmink M, et al. A randomized prospective study on the treatment of intra-articular distal radius fractures: open reduction and internal fixation with dorsal plating versus mini open reduction, percutaneous fixation, and external fixation. J Hand Surg Am 2005;30(4):764–72.
6. Kapoor H, Agarwal A, Dhaon BK. Displaced intra-articular fractures of distal radius: a comparative evaluation of results following closed reduction, external fixation and open reduction with internal fixation. Injury 2000;31(2):75–9.
7. Kreder HJ, Hanel DP, Agel J, et al. Indirect reduction and percutaneous fixation versus open reduction and internal fixation for displaced intra-articular fractures of the distal radius: a randomised, controlled trial. J Bone Joint Surg Br 2005;87(6):829–36.
8. Wright TW, Horodyski M, Smith DW. Functional outcome of unstable distal radius fractures: ORIF with a volar fixed-angle tine plate versus external fixation. J Hand Surg Am 2005;30(2):289–99.
9. Hutchinson DT, Bachus KN, Higgenbotham T. External fixation of the distal radius: to predrill or not to predrill. J Hand Surg Am 2000;25(6):1064–8.
10. Moroni A, Vannini F, Mosca M, et al. State of the art review: techniques to avoid pin loosening and

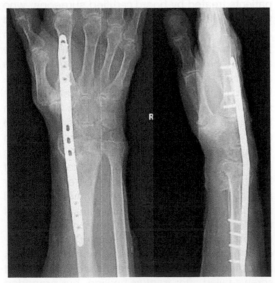

Fig. 2. Broken plate 5 months after bridge plate fixation of a distal radius fracture in an 85-year-old woman. The patient had bilateral distal radius fractures, and the distraction plates used for fixation broke in the same location.

infection in external fixation. J Orthop Trauma 2002; 16(3):189–95.

11. Anderson JT, Lucas GL, Buhr BR. Complications of treating distal radius fractures with external fixation: a community experience. Iowa Orthop J 2004;24:53–9.

12. Atroshi I, Brogren E, Larsson GU, et al. Wrist-bridging versus non-bridging external fixation for displaced distal radius fractures: a randomized assessor-blind clinical trial of 38 patients followed for 1 year. Acta Orthop 2006;77(3):445–53.

13. Harley BJ, Scharfenberger A, Beaupre LA, et al. Augmented external fixation versus percutaneous pinning and casting for unstable fractures of the distal radius—a prospective randomized trial. J Hand Surg Am 2004;29(5):815–24.

14. Hutchinson DT, Strenz GO, Cautilli RA. Pins and plaster vs external fixation in the treatment of unstable distal radial fractures. A randomized prospective study. J Hand Surg Br 1995;20(3):365–72.

15. Leung F, Tu YK, Chew WY, et al. Comparison of external and percutaneous pin fixation with plate fixation for intra-articular distal radial fractures. A randomized study. J Bone Joint Surg Am 2008; 90(1):16–22.

16. Krishnan J, Wigg AE, Walker RW, et al. Intra-articular fractures of the distal radius: a prospective randomised controlled trial comparing static bridging and dynamic non-bridging external fixation. J Hand Surg Br 2003;28(5):417–21.

17. McQueen MM, Hajducka C, Court-Brown CM. Redisplaced unstable fractures of the distal radius: a prospective randomised comparison of four methods of treatment. J Bone Joint Surg Br 1996; 78(3):404–9.

18. Raskin KB, Melone CP Jr. Unstable articular fractures of the distal radius. Comparative techniques of ligamentotaxis. Orthop Clin North Am 1993; 24(2):275–86.

19. Sanders RA, Keppel FL, Waldrop JI. External fixation of distal radial fractures: results and complications. J Hand Surg Am 1991;16(3):385–91.

20. Sommerkamp TG, Seeman M, Silliman J, et al. Dynamic external fixation of unstable fractures of the distal part of the radius. A prospective, randomized comparison with static external fixation. J Bone Joint Surg Am 1994;76(8):1149–61.

21. Werber KD, Raeder F, Brauer RB, et al. External fixation of distal radial fractures: four compared with five pins: a randomized prospective study. J Bone Joint Surg Am 2003;85(4):660–6.

22. Hanel DP, Lu TS, Weil WM. Bridge plating of distal radius fractures: the Harborview method. Clin Orthop Relat Res 2006;445:91–9.

23. Ruch DS, Ginn TA, Yang CC, et al. Use of a distraction plate for distal radial fractures with metaphyseal and diaphyseal comminution. J Bone Joint Surg Am 2005;87(5):945–54.

24. Ginn TA, Ruch DS, Yang CC, et al. Use of a distraction plate for distal radial fractures with metaphyseal and diaphyseal comminution. J Bone Joint Surg Am 2006;88(Suppl 1 Pt 1):29–36.

25. Wolf JC, Weil WM, Hanel DP, et al. A biomechanic comparison of an internal radiocarpal-spanning 2.4-mm locking plate and external fixation in a model of distal radius fractures. J Hand Surg Am 2006; 31(10):1578–86.

26. Agee JM. Distal radius fractures. Multiplanar ligamentotaxis. Hand Clin 1993;9(4):577–85.

27. Weber SC, Szabo RM. Severely comminuted distal radial fracture as an unsolved problem: complications associated with external fixation and pins and plaster techniques. J Hand Surg [Am] 1986;11(2):157–65.

Distal Radius Instability and Stiffness: Common Complications of Distal Radius Fractures

William B. Kleinman, MD[a,b,*]

KEYWORDS

• Distal radius fractures • Distal radio-ulna joint
• Instability • Stiffness

There is a plethora of peer reviewed journal articles, manuscripts, and book chapters in the hand surgical and general orthopedic literature on methods of treating distal radius fractures. The overwhelming majority of these writings focus on providing guidance to treating surgeons for making the most appropriate choices needed to realign displaced distal radius fracture fragments and to re-establish painless function of the upper limb after trauma-induced fractures of the distal radius. Most investigators focus on the importance of articular congruity and alignment, emphasizing the critical nature of the articular support surface for the carpus. It is presumed that only with meticulous realignment of joint surface anatomy is long-term, healthy carpal mechanics possible. Until the 2 most recent decades, however, little emphasis has been placed on the great morbidity and compromise to upper limb function that is associated with distal radioulnar joint (DRUJ) pathology occurring with fractures of the distal radius.[1–3] Emphasis, however, in the literature regarding distal radius fracture management over the past hundred years has been on restoration of anatomic radiocarpal alignment. The premise of this article is emphasizing to treating surgeons that the attention they give to restoration of anatomy of the DRUJ should be considered at least as important as the attention given to the radiocarpal relationship.

For more than 100 years, practicing clinicians have understood that forearm rotation (not radiocarpal flexion/extension or radioulnar deviation) is the critical movement of the upper limb that enables the hand to be put or placed advantageously in space, into positions that most maximize the ability of the hand to perform work (**Fig. 1**). DRUJ health is critical to the effectiveness of hand function. In extreme cases of distal radius fracture where resultant painful traumatic arthritis of the radiocarpal joint threatens effective hand function, arthrodesis of the wrist can eliminate pain, provide stability, and restore effective use of the hand. Contrary to this, painful traumatic arthritis of the DRUJ resulting from severe fracture extension through the sigmoid fossa severely compromises forearm rotation by stiffness and pain, leading to incapacitating dysfunction of the entire upper limb. The ability to effectively put or place the hand in space has been lost. Without healthy, painless, and stable forearm rotation, limb function is lost; substitution of combined shoulder/elbow kinematics is inadequate to compensate for the stiff forearm. Function of the

[a] The Indiana Hand to Shoulder Center, 8501 Harcourt Road, Indianapolis, IN 46260, USA
[b] Department of Orthopaedic Surgery, Indiana University School of Medicine, 541 Clinical Drive #600, Indianapolis, IN 46202, USA
* The Indiana Hand to Shoulder Center, 8501 Harcourt Road, Indianapolis, IN 46260.
E-mail address: WBK@Hand.MD

Hand Clin 26 (2010) 245–264
doi:10.1016/j.hcl.2010.01.004

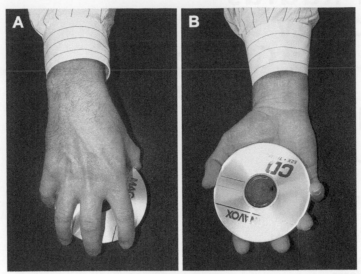

Fig. 1. Rotation of the forearm is critical for putting or placing the hand in space for maximum function (*A*,*B*).

limb would be severely inhibited by DRUJ arthrodesis.[4–6]

In spite of this common awareness, too little attention has been focused on the DRUJ in treating fractures of the distal radius. As discussed in this article, the energy of injury can result in fracture comminution that extends into the sigmoid fossa (resulting in significant displacement and disruption of DRUJ mechanics), axial compression, and shortening of the distal radius relative to the ulna, resulting in ulnar-plus variance,[7] or into the guidance mechanism for forearm rotation between distal radius and ulna by damage to the triangular fibrocartilage (TFC). This article also points out how stiffness of forearm rotation can result from a well-treated distal radius fracture and how this function-compromising complication can be effectively treated to restore healthy upper limb function.

BASIC ANATOMY

The seat of the distal ulna is a fulcrum around which all distal forearm movement and mechanics take place (freedom of rotation of the radial head at the proximal radioulnar joint [PRUJ] of the elbow is critical to normal forearm mechanics; because this article is focused on pathology of the distal radius, only the DRUJ is considered). In the bipedal human condition, the radius/carpus/hand unit rests squarely on this fulcrum, with gravity and an extrinsic extensor and flexor muscle load pulling the sigmoid fossa (the DRUJ contact area of the radius) securely against the seat of the ulna in neutral forearm rotation.[1–3]

In neutral rotation, the radius/carpus/hand unit sits squarely on the fulcrum provided by the ulnar seat. In equilibrium, the load borne by the hand (*F*) multiplied by the distance of this load from the DRUJ fulcrum (*L*) must equal the force required to stabilize the radial head at the PRUJ (*F'*) multiplied by the length of the entire forearm (*L'*) (**Fig. 2**). Therefore, in equilibrium, $F \times L = F' \times L'$. The total load borne by the DRUJ fulcrum (the seat of the ulna) is referred to as the joint reaction force (JRF) (**Fig. 3**). This JRF is equal to the sum of the moments ($F \times L$) on both the distal and proximal sides of the DRUJ fulcrum. Therefore, the DRUJ JRF = $F \times L + F' \times L'$ (**Fig. 4**). The JRF at

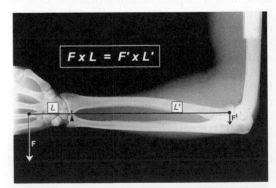

$$F \times L = F' \times L'$$

Fig. 2. In equilibrium, the moments on the distal and proximal sides of the ulnar seat fulcrum must be equal. The load in the hand (F) times the distance of the load from the fulcrum (L) must be equal to the length of the forearm from the fulcrum (L') times the resistance to displacement provided by the annular ligament at the radial head (F').

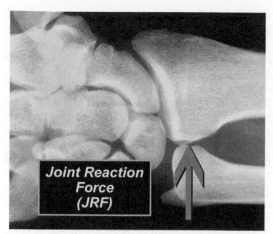

Fig. 3. The seat of the ulna is the fulcrum for all DRUJ mechanics. Because most upper limb activities in the bipedal human occur with the radiocarpal unit "on top" of the ulnar seat, the JRF at the DRUJ can be enormous. The JRF is proportional to the load in the hand, the force of all muscles acting to pull the radius and ulna together for stability, and the force of gravity acting on the hand/forearm unit.

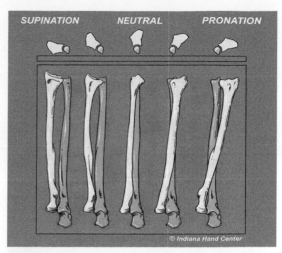

Fig. 5. As the radius rotates from full supination to full pronation around a nonrotating, fixed ulna, the radiocarpal unit shortens relative to the ulna, resulting in ulnar-plus variance in the pronated position. (*Courtesy of* The Indiana Hand to Shoulder Center.)

the DRUJ can be enormous, easily 6 to 8 times body weight.

The ulna does not participate in actual rotation of the forearm. It is fixed to the humerus at the ginglymus ulnotrochlear joint. The ulna flexes and extends at the elbow but does not rotate. All forearm rotation involves a pivoting motion of the radius/carpus/hand unit from a position parallel to the ulna in full forearm supination to a crossover position of the radius relative to the ulna in full pronation (**Fig. 5**). Because the ulna is fixed with respect to forearm rotation, the radius shortens relative to the fixed ulna length as it crosses over the ulna into pronation.

As the radial head at the PRUJ rotates around the fixed, longitudinal axis of rotation, the sigmoid fossa of the distal radius rotates and translates relative to the fixed seat of the ulna. In full supination, the principal axis of load bearing (the principal axis is an engineering term used to define an imaginary point at the center of an infinite number of cluster points between 2 loaded surfaces in contact with each other) between sigmoid fossa and ulnar seat is volar and proximal.

In full forearm pronation, with radius crossed over the ulna (and relatively shortened), the principal axis of load bearing is at the dorsal and distal margin of the sigmoid fossa. Thus, through a full arc of forearm rotation, the center of contact points on the articular surfaces of the sigmoid fossa and ulnar seat forms a tracking line along the fossa, from proximal-volar in supination to distal-dorsal in pronation (**Fig. 6**).

Long-term health of the diarthrodial DRUJ is based on cartilage integrity and anatomic structures that guide the radius around the ulna from full supination to full pronation. Surface cartilage thrives under conditions of physiologic compression.

In cases of intra-articular injury to the DRUJ created by distal radius fracture, resultant step-off deformity generates surface shear forces at the DRUJ causing chondrolysis, which predisposes the joint to traumatic arthritis. The best efforts at anatomic alignment of displaced intra-articular DRUJ fracture fragments are to reduce this propensity toward painful traumatic arthritis that

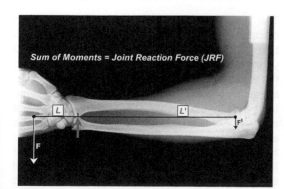

Fig. 4. The sum of the moments on the distal and proximal sides of the fulcrum equals the JRF at the DRUJ.

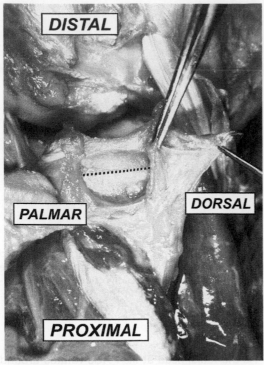

DISTAL

PALMAR

DORSAL

PROXIMAL

Fig. 6. The principal axis of load-bearing tracks across the sigmoid fossa from proximal/volar in supination to distal/dorsal in pronation.

predictably results from step-off deformity and loss of DRUJ cartilage, secondary to shear forces.

DRUJ stability through a full arc of pronosupination is provided by extrinsic structures arising proximal to the distal end of the ulna and intrinsic structures at the distal end of the ulna itself. Extrinsic stabilizers contribute DRUJ guidance to a minor degree. They consist of (1) the extensor carpi ulnaris tendon (ECU), (2) the sixth dorsal compartment subsheath for the ECU,[8,9] (3) the superficial and deep heads of the pronator quadratus muscle,[10] and (4) the interosseous ligament.[11]

Much more significant for providing DRUJ stability through its physiologic arc of pronosupination is its intrinsic stabilizer, the TFC.[1–3,12–21] This small, architecturally complicated piece of connective tissue is critical for normal DRUJ mechanics. Among other components (**Fig. 7**), the TFC consists of deep and superficial peripheral portions, coursing along its dorsal and volar margins. These peripheral fibrous portions of the TFC are well vascularized.[14,15] They attach the medial border of the distal ulna to the medial border of the distal radius and are also referred to as the dorsal and palmar limbi of the TFC. They are responsible for providing primary guidance to the radius/carpus/hand unit as it rotates

and translates around the fixed ulna (see **Figs. 5** and **6**).

Injuries to the peripheral TFC in association with distal radius fractures have the potential to disrupt the critical rotation/translation DRUJ guidance system, leading to painful ulnar-sided wrist instability and, if left untreated, shearing of the cartilage surfaces of the DRUJ and eventual traumatic arthritis. This predictable degeneration of joint surfaces can occur even with displaced, extra-articular distal radius fractures that do not involve fracture extension into the DRUJ articular surface. Articular congruity and DRUJ surface alignment are critical for long-term healthy function after trauma.

The most important component of the TFC for providing rotation/translation guidance for the radius/carpus/hand unit is the deep component, called the ligamentum subcruentum. This thick, strong, fibrous connective tissue arises at the well-vascularized fovea of the distal ulna and attaches to the medial volar and dorsal margins of the distal radius, just distal to the sigmoid fossa. Because of its wide angle of attachment from origin to insertion, the ligamentum subcruentum (dorsal and volar components) is more effective in providing guidance for rotation than the superficial components of the peripheral TFC, which originate from the more medial ulnar styloid, and blend together with the fibers of the ligamentum subcruentum on the medial, distal radius (**Fig. 8**). The well-vascularized superficial and deep components of the TFC envelope the poorly vascularized articular disc of the TFC, the central structure responsible for axial load transfer from the ulnar side of the carpus to the pole of the distal ulna (see **Fig. 7**).

CONSEQUENCES OF SUPRAPHYSIOLOGIC LOADS ON THE TFC IN ASSOCIATION WITH FRACTURES OF THE DISTAL RADIUS

The association of ulnar styloid fractures with distal radius fractures has been observed even before the advent of radiographs more than 100 years ago. Although the mechanism of injury to the radius has been easy to reproduce (conceptually and in the laboratory), the mechanism of injury to the distal end of the ulna has been more of a mystery until the past 25 years. In 1990, Pogue and colleagues[22] published a landmark article from their laboratory data, shedding considerable light onto the black box of disorders at the distal end of the ulna. These researchers attempted to simulate extra-articular fractures of the distal radius by removing a variety of metaphyseal cadaver bone sections and observing whether or

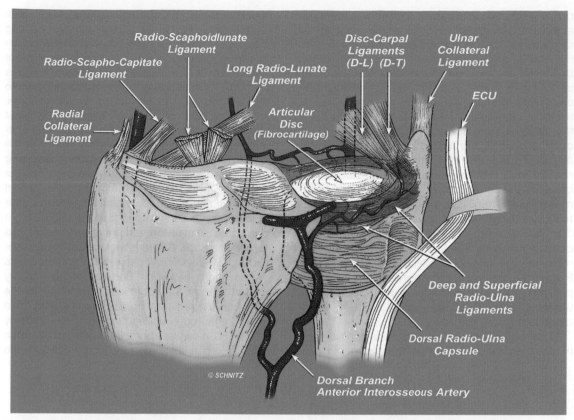

Fig. 7. The primary intrinsic stabilizer of the DRUJ is the TFC. The TFC complex consists of superficial (*green*) and deep (*blue*) radioulnar fibers, the 2 disc-carpal ligaments (disc-lunate and disc-triquetral), and the central articular disc (*white*). The articular disc is responsible for load transfer from the medial carpus to the pole of the distal ulna, particularly in ulnar deviation. The vascularized, peripheral radioulnar ligaments (*green and blue*) are nourished by dorsal and palmar branches of the posterior interosseous artery, and are responsible for guiding the radiocarpal unit around the seat of the ulna. (*Courtesy of* The Indiana Hand to Shoulder Center.)

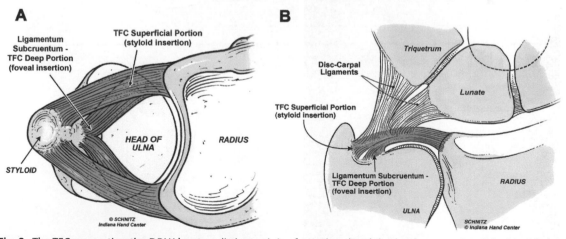

Fig. 8. The TFC supporting the DRUJ has two distinct origins from the ulna (*A*). The deep portion (*blue*) is referred to as the ligamentum subcruentum and originates from the fovea, just medial to the articular surface of the ulnar pole. The superficial portion (*green*) originates from the base of the ulna styloid. These 2 independent insertions allow different components of the TFC to tighten in different positions of forearm rotation (*B*). The angles of origin to insertion of these 2 components of the TFC are quite different, making the deep, blue fibers (ligamentum subcruentum) considerably more effective as a DRUJ stabilizer through the full arc of forearm pronosupination. (*Courtesy of* The Indiana Hand to Shoulder Center.)

not the remaining fragments of radius could be apposed without osteotomizing the ulnar styloid through its base (the components of the TFC remained intact). The investigators demonstrated that they could shorten the distal radius 2 mm and 4 mm and still bring the remaining bone segments together securely without releasing the tethering effect of an intact TFC by cutting through the base of the ulnar styloid. Similarly, they were able to change the inclination of the radiocarpal articular surface to 10° and the tilt of the distal radius to 0°, both without cutting through the base of the ulnar styloid. Shortening the radius more than 4 mm, changing the radius inclination to 0°, and creating a dorsal radius tilt of 15° or 30°, however, were all unachievable without first cutting through the ulnar styloid base, thus relieving the tethering effect of the intact TFC. Pogue and colleagues[22] theorized, "Severely displaced distal radius fractures not displaying an ulnar styloid fracture might have a TFCC disruption."

The implications of this work are considerable: in vivo, as the distal radius fails from the usual mechanism of fall on the outstretched hand; supraphysiologic forces surpass the load-bearing capacity of the bone. The bone fractures (shortening, collapsing dorsally, tilting radially, or a combination) as sudden and extreme force is propagated through the bone and farther on into the TFC through the limbi of its peripheral fibers. If displacement of fracture fragments is great enough, then the connective tissue of the TFC itself will fail (resulting in a peripheral tear) or the kinetic energy dissipated by the failing, collapsing distal radius will continue along its path of least resistance (the intact TFC) into the ulnar styloid (**Fig. 9**). If the energy bolus is sufficient to cause displacement of the radius fracture fragments, it can cause an avulsion fracture of the ulnar styloid through its base. Basilar styloid fractures in association with displaced fractures of the distal radius are common; they occur because of the anatomy of the origin of the superficial component of the TFC from the proximal portion of the styloid.[1–3]

With a thorough understanding of the anatomy of the TFC, it can be appreciated that if an avulsion fracture of the ulnar styloid occurs (via extreme

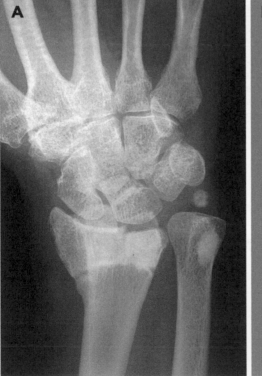
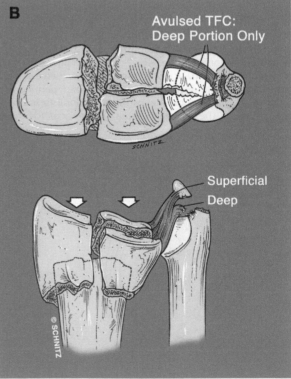

Fig. 9. Anteroposterior radiograph (*A*) and artist rendering (*B*) of the effect of a distal radius fracture on the TFC. Displacement or shortening of the distal radius transmits forces through the tethering TFC, tearing the superficial and deep fibers from their respective origins (styloid and fovea, respectively) or avulsing the ulnar styloid from its base, with tearing of the deep ligamentum subcruentum from its foveal origin. Shortening and fragment collapse of the distal radius must be significant enough to affect the TFC. (*Courtesy of* The Indiana Hand to Shoulder Center.)

tension on the superficial TFC from a collapsing distal radius fracture) and if the ulnar styloid is displaced, then—by definition—the deep fibers of the TFC (ligamentum subcruentum, originating at the fovea of the distal ulna) must also be torn from their origin. The degree of separation of the ligamentum subcruentum from its foveal origin must be equal to the degree of displacement of the ulnar styloid from its base (see **Fig. 9**). Because the superficial and deep components of the TFC run together intimately and insert together on the medial radius, separation of the fractured ulnar styloid from its base (with an intact superficial TFC component) must equal separation of the failed ligamentum subcruentum from its foveal origin.

Although the article by Pogue and colleagues[22] is important in providing insight into potential failure of TFC components in association with fractures of the distal radius, their work was only a laboratory simulation of radius trauma. It could not address inherent elasticity or stretchability of the tissue of the TFC itself. Is it fair or accurate to suggest that every displaced basilar styloid fracture must be associated with a complete separation of the ligamentum subcruentum from its foveal origin, resulting in DRUJ instability? In the clinical arena, the inherent elasticity of the peripheral components of the TFC must be taken into consideration when discussing why certain catastrophic failures of the distal radius are associated with neither styloid fracture nor TFC injury. But the work of Pogue and colleagues provides fuel for thought. In every case in which an avulsion basilar ulnar styloid fracture is observed, thought should be given to carefully examining the DRUJ relationship by a stress test of the joint under anesthesia (**Figs. 10** and **11**). The potential for DRUJ instability always exists if a displaced distal radius fracture is associated with a basilar ulnar styloid fracture.

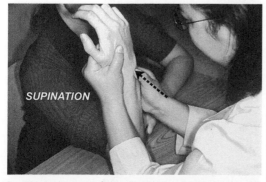

Fig. 10. Stress test of the dorsal, deep fibers of the ligamentum subcruentum for pain, mechanical instability, or both (findings must be compared with the opposite, uninjured side).

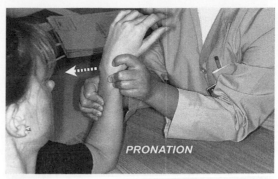

Fig. 11. Stress test of the volar, deep fibers of the ligament subcruentum for pain, mechanical instability, or both (findings must be compared with the opposite, uninjured side).

Whether or not surgical attention should be paid to the TFC or the displaced ulnar styloid fracture should be based on clinical findings obtained by examination under anesthesia. The following are guidelines I have used for many years to establish criteria for surgical management of the ulnar side of the wrist in cases of radius open reduction and internal fixation (ORIF) when the degree of initial radius fracture displacement suggests there should be legitimate concerns about DRUJ stability.

ALGORITHM FOR SURGICAL MANAGEMENT OF THE ULNAR SIDE OF THE WRIST IN ASSOCIATION WITH DISPLACED FRACTURES OF THE DISTAL RADIUS

Step 1: If a clinician thinks that indications are present for ORIF of a distal radius fracture for radiocarpal and DRUJ alignment, surgical stability of the radius must first be attained using whatever technique the surgeon thinks is in the best interest of the patient. **Fig. 12** shows severe fragment displacement requiring ligamentodesis plus percutaneous Kirschner (K)-wire fixation for alignment after application of a hand-forearm external fixator. In another example, **Fig. 13** shows rigid internal fixation achieved with a volar buttress locking plate and screws. DRUJ stability relies, then, predominately on the volar ligamentum subcruentum in pronation.

Step 2: With rigid stability of the distal radius fracture fragments achieved, a surgeon can stress test the stability of the DRUJ by fully supinating the forearm and trying to displace the distal ulna volarly. Full forearm supination renders the superficial volar fibers of the TFC ineffective, whereas stability relies almost entirely on the deep, dorsal fibers of the ligamentum subcruentum (**Fig. 14**). This provocative maneuver places supraphysiologic load on the dorsal fibers of the ligamentum

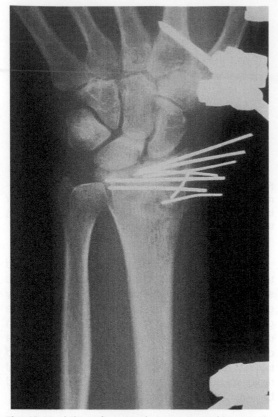

Fig. 12. Stability of a severely comminuted intra-articular distal radius fracture achieved by rigid external fixation and multiple percutaneous K-wire fixation. With radius stability achieved, the stability of the DRUJ can be tested by provocative maneuvers.

subcruentum, the most critical DRUJ stabilizer of the TFC in full supination. Landmark work published by Hagert in 1994[20] illustrates the importance of the deep fibers of the TFC when stressing the forearm in supination. Once a surgeon demonstrates any degree of DRUJ instability in supination, then the forearm can be pronated. As the sigmoid fossa of the radius translates volarly in pronation, the head of the ulna (seat and pole) moves under and outside the guidance control of the superficial dorsal TFC fibers (**Fig. 15**). Stress testing the volar fibers of the ligamentum subcruentum demonstrates how important this part of the TFC is in preventing supraphysiologic volar translation of the radius/carpus/hand (see **Fig. 14**).

Consider rupture of the entire peripheral origin of the TFC, except for the thinnest, yet intact portion of the volar ligamentum subcruentum. As the forearm is rotated into pronation, and the radius/carpus/hand unit passively translated volarly on the ulnar seat, the DRUJ will still be stable. As the examining surgeon rotates and translates the forearm into supination, however, injury to the dorsal ligamentum subcruentum will allow the sigmoid fossa to translate dorsally off the seat of the ulna, resulting in gross DRUJ instability in supination. Similarly, if there has been rupture of the entire TFC in association with the displaced distal radius fracture, but a thin portion of the dorsal ligamentum subcruentum remains intact, then, although passive supination of the forearm reveals the DRUJ to be stable, there would be gross instability in pronation (ie, supraphysiologic volar translation of the sigmoid fossa relative to the ulnar seat).

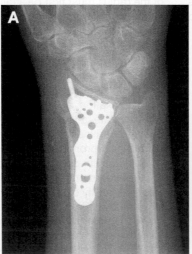
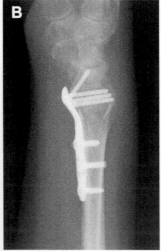

Fig. 13. (A–B) AP and lateral x-rays showing rigid internal or external fixation of a displaced distal radius fracture (in this case, by Acu Loc plate and screws) affords the surgeon an opportunity to stress test the integrity of the components of the TFC.

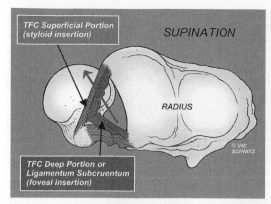

Fig. 14. An illustration of tightening of the dorsal, deep fibers of the ligamentum subcruentum as the radius rotates and translates dorsally off the seat of the ulna in supination. The head of the ulna translates along the sigmoid fossa, and herniates out from under cover of tightening superficial palmar TFC fibers, rendering these fibers ineffective in controlling DRUJ mechanics. (*Courtesy of* The Indiana Hand to Shoulder Center.)

If the TFC has been completely avulsed from the ulnar fovea and from the intact ulnar styloid (complete failure of deep and superficial fibers), then the DRUJ will be globally unstable when stress tested in pronation and supination. These also are the findings with complete foveal avulsion of the ligamentum subcruentum and a displaced fracture through the base of the ulnar styloid (see **Fig. 9**).

Step 3: The surgeon should next put on an extra pair of sterile gloves and perform the same stress maneuvers on the undamaged, contralateral

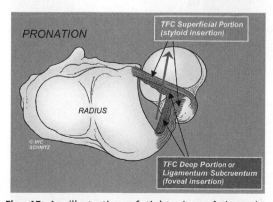

Fig. 15. An illustration of tightening of the volar, deep fibers of the ligamentum subcruentum as the radius rotates and translates palmarly off the seat of the ulna in pronation. The head of the ulna translates along the sigmoid fossa and herniates out from under cover of tightening superficial dorsal TFC fibers, rendering these fibers relatively ineffective in controlling DRUJ mechanics. (*Courtesy of* The Indiana Hand to Shoulder Center.)

forearm, sensing any differences in stability between the normal and injured sides.

When continuing to acquire information about the integrity of the TFC with a distal radius fracture that has required ORIF, surgeons should be cognizant of the important laboratory work by af Ekenstam and colleagues in 1984 and 1985[13,18] regarding DRUJ instability with simulated distal radius fracture malunion and intact TFC components. Extra-articular malunions of the distal radius resulting from poorly reduced or inadequately fixed distal radius fractures are notorious for demonstrating concomitant DRUJ instability, even with the TFC uninjured. Not only is the radiocarpal articular surface malaligned, predisposing to many pathologic conditions, including carpal instability,[23] and not only is the tracking line for the principal axis of load bearing at the DRUJ improperly oriented for healthy mechanics (predisposing the DRUJ to cartilage breakdown from surface shear over time) but also the capacity of the dorsal limbi of the peripheral TFC to stabilize pronosupination of the radius/carpus/hand around the ulnar seat is rendered ineffective by the dorsal collapse of the distal radius malunion. The cadaver work of af Ekenstam and Hagert[24] simulates structural changes in TFC alignment with radius malunions of 30° dorsal tilt. The investigators demonstrate how—with an intact TFC—the DRUJ can appear grossly unstable as the sigmoid fossa translates and rolls dorsally off the ulnar seat. The fossa itself is no longer mechanically able to contain the ulnar seat, and the orientation of the dorsal fibers of the TFC in cases of malunion allows the seat of the ulna to seem to subluxate against the volar capsule of the DRUJ. The appearance is suggestive of an ineffective checkrein effect of the volar ligamentum subcruentum, but, in cases of dorsal malunion, collapse of the dorsal radius without TFC injury of any kind can allow the seat of the ulna to supraphysiologically translate volar relative to the sigmoid fossa.[24]

Step 4: Demonstrable DRUJ instability associated with the distal radius fracture and coexistence of a basilar displaced ulnar styloid fracture indicate not only that energy introduced into the system by the injury has pulled off the styloid via the superficial peripheral fibers of the TFC but also, by definition, the ligamentum subcruentum has been avulsed from the fovea, leading to gross instability. By anatomically reducing the ulnar styloid by ORIF (**Fig. 16**), not only is the tension of the superficial TFC restored to normal but also the critical, injured ligamentum subcruentum is restored as closely as anatomically possible to the fovea, allowing for primary healing to take place at its origin.

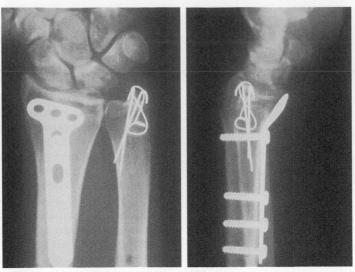

Fig. 16. Anteroposterior and lateral postoperative radiographs of a 36-year-old man who fell on his outstretched hand, resulting in a closed, comminuted extra-articular distal radius fracture, with avulsion of the ulnar styloid by an intact superficial component of the TFC. Once anatomic reduction of the radius was secured by rigid plating, an ORIF of the ulnar styloid was anatomically achieved by tension band wiring. This technique brings the ligamentum subcruentum back to its site of foveal origin for healing.

The literature on the subject remains contradictory and controversial; but personal experience suggest a strong indication for restoration of bony anatomy, if the basilar ulna styloid fracture fragment is displaced more than 2 mms.

Step 5: If there is demonstrable instability (relative to the contralateral side) but no fracture of the ulnar styloid, then there has to have been a substantial tear through the periphery of the TFC itself. In these cases, the TFC must be repaired or reattached to the ulnar fovea to avoid chronic DRUJ instability once the distal radius has healed and the patient rehabilitated. If an external fixator has been used to stabilize the radius fracture, then triangulation of the fixator to the ulna obviates cast immobilization (**Fig. 17**). With more common use of volar locking plates and other plate fixation devices over the past decade, I have replaced frame triangulation with the simple external fixation provided by percutaneous pins and long-arm cast, which minimize the risks of subtle and inadvertent pronosupination during the 6-week TFC healing period. **Fig. 18** shows a simple K-wire and wire-loop technique of ORIF of the ulnar styloid. **Fig. 19** shows placement of two 0.062-in percutaneous K-wires with a bone anchor used to restore the anatomy of an avulsed ligamentum subcruentum. **Fig. 20** shows the sequence of steps used in implanting a bone anchor and sutures into the ulnar fovea, securing the TFC to its original place of origin. In 2009, Souer and colleagues[25] published their level III research study of the effect of an unrepaired

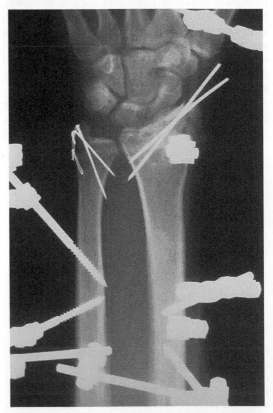

Fig. 17. Hand-forearm rigid external fixation (radius to second metacarpal) can be triangulated to the ulna to rigidly hold the forearm bones in neutral rotation while the injured ligamentum subcruentum heals.

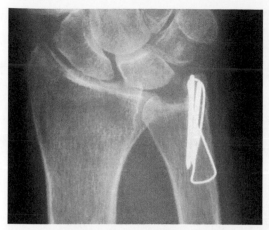

Fig. 18. Tension band wiring of an avulsed ulnar styloid fracture is technically not demanding and allows predictable styloid and ligamentum subcruentum healing, avoiding DRUJ instability.

fracture of the ulna styloid base on patient outcomes after plate-and-screw fixation of a distal radial fracture. Two coherts of seventy-six matched patients were used for their study. The authors concluded no significant differences

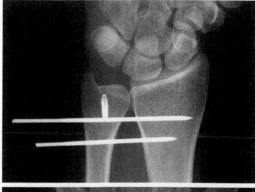

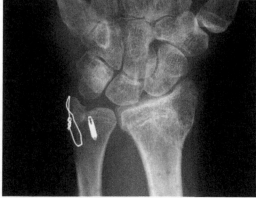

Fig. 19. Two examples of bone anchors placed deep into the fovea. Attached sutures grasp the ligamentum subcruentum, pulling it deep into its foveal origin for healing.

were found between patients with unrepaired fractures of the styloid base and those with no ulnar styloid fracture. Styloid fracture displacements were greater than 2 mm.

In 2009, Sameer and colleagues[26] reported on a 5-year cohort of patients subjected to the Michigan Hand Outcomes Questionnaire (MHOQ). Each patient had undergone ORIF of a displaced distal radius fracture. Each had a concomitant ulnar styloid fracture. The interest of the investigators was whether or not ORIF of the concommitant ulnar styloid fracture affected the subjective outcome of treatment. The background of their work was a century of clinical studies that have been inconclusive about the relationship of chronic DRUJ instability and displacement of a fractured ulnar styloid. They concluded that patients with DRUJ instability post ORIF of a displaced distal radius fracture did not benefit subjectively from ORIF of the displaced distal ulnar styloid fracture. Outcomes seemed to be similar whether or not the styloid was fixed.[26]

Jupiter and colleagues, also in 2009,[27] corroborated the work of Chung and colleagues, by suggesting, in a retrospective review of their two cohorts of 76 matched patients, that the displaced ulnar styloid, in association with a displaced distal radius fracture, does not have to be fixed to achieve a good outcome.

There are important questions to be asked about the conclusions of these works. First, regarding the article by Chung and colleagues, is the MHOQ an appropriate measuring tool for assessment of the chronic DRUJ instability dilemma? Second, has any of the patients studied in either report experienced a displaced basilar styloid fracture? And third, how is postradius fixation DRUJ instability measured intraoperatively? Is it precise? Is it consistent?

Commentary by Jupiter[28] on the 2009 work by Chung and colleagues[25] suggests the importance of fibers of the distal oblique bundle of the interosseous membrane (IOM) in preventing DRUJ instability. Jupiter defines instability only in gross terms: the piano key sign or the palpable clunk of the medial radius rolling off the seat of the ulna at the end arc of pronation or supination. I consider this definition of DRUJ instability is an oversimplification. DRUJ instability is a spectrum of pathologic laxity at the distal end of the ulna, ranging from microinstability demonstrated only by provocative maneuvers that cause pain to gross mechanical instability alluded to by Jupiter in his commentary. Whether or not the distal oblique fibers of the IOM are intact, it is an anatomic fact that displacement of a basilar ulnar styloid fracture cannot occur without rupture or significant

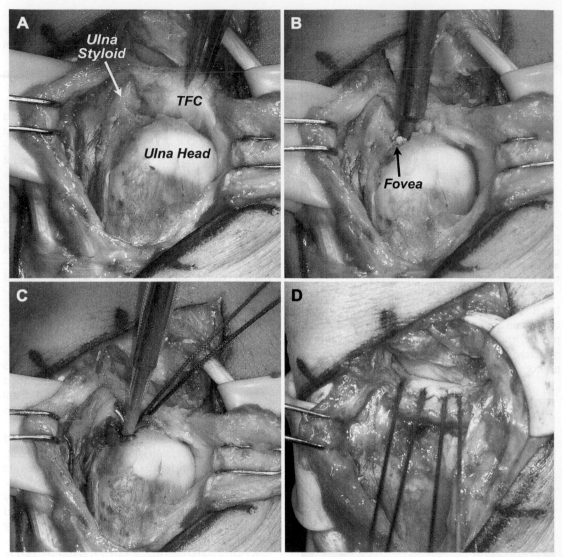

Fig. 20. (*A*) the exposed components of the distal end of the ulna; (*B–C*) once placed deeply into the fovea, the standard 2-0 suture material manufactured with the anchor can be reinforced by the surgeon by adding additional suture material to the anchor, giving a potential 4-strand attachment of the avulsed, deep radioulnar fibers of the ligamentum subcruentum to bone; (*D*) the final position of sutures prior to the ligamentum subcruentum being tied securely to the ulna fovea. Currently, many companies manufacture two 4-strand bone-anchors of appropriate size.

attention of this origin of the ligamentum subcruentum (deep TFC fibers, primarily responsible for DRUJ stability) from their foveal attachment, independent of the TFC origin from the ulnar styloid itself.

Although I agree with the authors'[25,26] assessment of middle- and distal-third styloid fractures, extensive clinical experience and intimate knowledge of the anatomy of TFC suggest strong indications for ORIF of the displaced basilar styloid fracture. Failure to do so can lead to chronic, painful DRUJ instability. For these reasons, I continue

to teach my fellows and recommend to my patients ORIF of basilar styloid fractures when in association with displaced distal radius fractures requiring ORIF. DRUJ instability should always be suspected preoperatively and demonstrated with a stress test intraoperatively.

In 1991, I published experience of reattaching the damaged periphery of the TFC to the ulnar styloid in chronic cases of painful instability after delayed treatment for trauma.[28] Since then, there have been 2 important developments: (1) appreciation of the anatomy of the TFC has evolved to

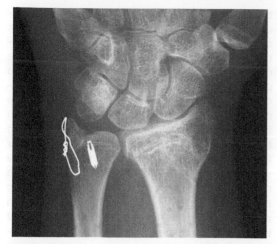

Fig. 21. Long-term follow-up anteroposterior radiograph. The patient recovered full, painless pronation/supination under load.

a better understanding of the dominance of the deep, foveal origin of the TFC (ligamentum subcruentum) in providing the primary guidance system at the DRUJ for pronosupination[2] and (2) the development of bone anchors to assure excellent fixation of the avulsed ligamentum subcruentum to the fovea (see Fig. 20; Fig. 21), rather than to a more peripheral position with sutures through the ulnar styloid, as I described 20 years ago. The beauty of the current use of bone anchors to reattach the avulsed TFC to the fovea (performed in conjunction with ORIF of fracture of the distal radius) is that reconstitution of stable, painless forearm pronosupination can be assured by direct and secure fixation of the TFC to an anatomic point now considered the critical origin of the TFC guidance system for the radius/carpus/hand unit.

CONSEQUENCES OF FAILING TO APPRECIATE TFC ANATOMY WHEN TREATING DISPLACED DISTAL RADIUS FRACTURES

An example of the consequences of failure to respect all components of these severe distal radius fractures, with potential for disturbance of normal DRUJ mechanics, is illustrated as follows. A 19-year-old female college student fell off her bicycle onto her outstretched dominant hand, incurring a grossly displaced, extra-articular distal radius fracture (Fig. 22). The extent of shortening and dorsal angulation is clear. Also readily seen is significant displacement of the ulnar styloid, avulsed through its base by an intact superficial radioulnar component of the TFC. The patient was treated elsewhere by closed reduction and cast immobilization until healed clinically and radiographically (Fig. 23). She presented for a second opinion at my office 9 months after her initial treatment (Fig. 24), complaining of disabling pain at the distal end of the ulna, particularly at the end arcs of loaded pronation and supination. Physical examination revealed (1) subtle hypermobility at the sigmoid fossa on a stress test of the ligamentum subcruentum, using the provocative maneuvers (described previously) shown in Figs. 10 and 11 (relative to the opposite side). The patient had full pronation and supination and 65° wrist extension/75° wrist flexion. There was no tenderness on direct palpation of the ulnar styloid fracture nonunion. The piano key sign was negative.

Radiographs of this young woman show a 6-mm, radially displaced malunion of the distal radius, with a 6-mm displacement of her ulnar styloid, avulsed through its bony base by the superficial dorsal and palmar radioular components of the TFC (see Fig. 24). The ulnar styloid has been displaced from its base exactly the

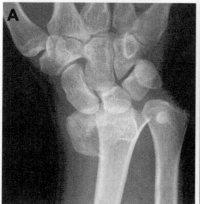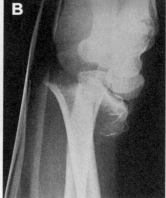

Fig. 22. Anterposterior (A) and lateral (B) radiographs of a 19-year-old woman who fell off a bicycle onto her outstretched dominant hand. The magnitude of radius shortening, dorsal angulation, and complete loss of inclination is readily seen.

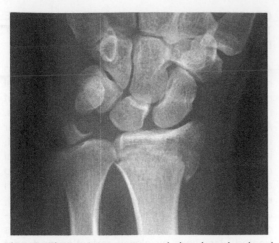

Fig. 23. The patient was treated elsewhere by closed reduction and cast immobilization for 6 weeks. Anteroposterior radiographs out of plaster reveal lateral displacement of the distal radius fragment, with similar lateral displacement of the ulnar styloid through its base, avulsed by the intact superficial radioulnar ligaments of the TFC.

same millimeter distance as the lateral displacement of the distal radius malunion. The original injury displacement of the distal radius fracture pulled the ulnar styloid from its base the same distance by force transmission through the intact superficial dorsal and palmar components of the TFC. As the bony styloid was avulsed from its base, the deep foveal attachments of the ligamentum subcruentum failed as well, destabilizing the DRUJ by loss of its critical anchor point. Failure by the first treating surgeon to anatomically reduce

the distal radius not only resulted in a radius malunion and ulnar styloid nonunion (see **Fig. 23**) but also left the avulsed fibers of origin of the ligamentum subcruentum directly on top of the hyaline cartilage of the distal ulnar pole. There was no potential whatsoever for the ligamentum subcruentum to heal to the fovea because of the magnitude of the initial fracture displacement. In this patient, failure of the ligamentum subcruentum to heal properly to its anatomic origin at the ulnar fovea resulted in chronic, painful DRUJ instability under load. The patient's 6-mm radius malunion not only shifted the ulnar styloid from its anatomic base but also left the ligamentum subcruentum displaced to a position from which it could not be reanchored to the fovea without corrective osteotomy of the radius.

A dome osteotomy of the radius was performed (**Fig. 25**), allowing a 6-mm medial shift of the distal radius along with the superficial radioulnar ligaments and articular disc, all still attached to the ulnar styloid. The restored anatomy of the radius then allowed the ulnar styloid fibrous union to be taken down, reduced, and anchored anatomically to its base using a tension band wiring technique. With the ulnar styloid anatomically reduced, the ligamentum subcruentum could be restored to its anatomic origin at the ulnar fovea with a bone anchor and sutures (see **Fig. 25**).

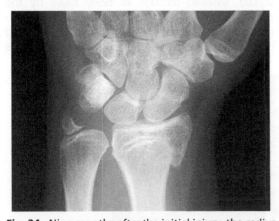

Fig. 24. Nine months after the initial injury, the radius is healed. The displaced ulnar styloid fracture nonunion is ankylosed and nontender, but the DRUJ is painful and unstable through a full arc of pronation/supination. Provocative maneuvers that stress the deep dorsal and deep palmar fibers of the ligamentum subcruentum were positive for pain and instability.

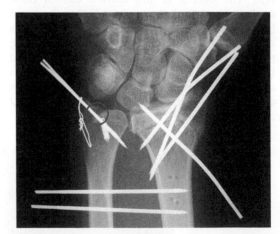

Fig. 25. Dome osteotomy of the radius malunion allowed a 6-mm medial shift of the distal radius fragment in this patient. The ulnar styloid could then be anatomically reduced at its base and held with tension band wires. With the bony anatomy restored, the critical, deep radioulnar ligaments of the ligamentum subcruentum were now juxtaposed to the fovea (*circle*) and could be securely reattached with a bone anchor. To eliminate any forearm rotation for 6 weeks, two 0.062-in K-wires were introduced percutaneously through the distal shaft of the ulna into the radius.

The critical concept in treating this case effectively was to shift the entire distal forearm unit medially, enabling anatomic restoration of the ligamentum subcruentum to the fovea and restoration of normal DRUJ mechanics. **Fig. 20** illustrates the intraoperative technique of preparing the fovea for reattachment of the ligamentum subcruentum, installing the bone anchor, and passing sutures through the TFC before pulling the deep fibers securely into the fovea. As seen in the postoperative radiograph (see **Fig. 25**), 2 additional percutaneous 0.062-in K-wires were passed through the distal ulna into the radius before tying the bone anchor sutures as tightly as possible in neutral forearm rotation. The K-wires maintain rigid stability of the DRUJ during early postoperative healing. All percutaneous K-wires seen in **Fig. 25** were removed 6 weeks after surgery. After rehabilitation, the patient regained full, painless pronosupination, with normal load-bearing capacity at the DRUJ. Her final radiograph is seen in **Fig. 21**.

OTHER DRUJ-DESTABILIZING INJURIES TO THE TFC IN ASSOCIATION WITH FRACTURE OF THE DISTAL RADIUS

The usual failure pattern of the TFC (as the radius fractures and collapses away from the intact ulna) is by peripheral tearing and separation of connective tissue fibers from their origin at the ulnar styloid or fovea or by an avulsion fracture of the ulnar styloid itself through its base (by the superficial TFC components).[1-3] As discussed previously, separation of the styloid from its base usually implies comcommitant separation of the ligamentum subcruentum origin at the fovea. Palmer[21] classified as type IB those peripheral TFC injuries that occur in the well-vascularized periphery; and, as the literature shows,[29] type IB TFC injuries are amenable to direct repair and healing. Repairs of peripheral tears of the TFC are now performed routinely, using an open or arthroscopic technique, based on the location and magnitude of the avulsion injury.

Palmer type IB tears of the TFC occur in the fibrous dorsal or volar portions connecting the medial distal ulna to the medial distal radius. Collagen fibers of this connective tissue have a transverse orientation from ulna origin to radius insertion. Microcirculation penetrates approximately 20% of the TFC dorsally and 20% volarly.[14,15] Nutrition of these portions of the TFC is entirely by its microcirculatory anatomy.

Palmer type IA lesions of the TFC involve the central articular disc, made up of fibrocartilageous tissue nourished by ulnocarpal synovial washing. Type IC lesions are rare and involve the disc-lunate or disc-triquetral volar components of the TFC. Palmer type ID injuries to the TFC involve separation of the TFC attachment to the medial border of the distal radius.

In my experience, acute type IA central injuries to the articular disc (the hypovascular, central portion of the TFC [see **Fig. 7**]) are rarely associated with displaced, distal radius fractures. Likewise, type IC failures of the volar disc-carpal ligaments (disc-lunate and disc-triquetral [see **Fig. 7**]) are also rare. More frequent (but still uncommon) are the type ID separations of the TFC insertion from the medial radius, in association with displaced distal radius fractures. Even with severe comminution and displacement of the medial column of the radius with intra-articular extension into the sigmoid fossa, a portion of the TFC attachment may be lost, but the bulk of the structure remains intact. In those unusual cases where there has been DRUJ instability rendered by TFC tearing from the medial border of the fractured radius, bone-anchor reattachment can be performed using open (or arthroscopic) techniques at the time of ORIF of the displaced distal radius fracture.

RESULTANT FOREARM STIFFNESS AFTER EFFECTIVE ORIF AND HEALING OF A DISPLACED DISTAL RADIUS FRACTURE

Forearm rotational stiffness is one of the most function-comprising consequences of wrist trauma. Although often painless, forearm stiffness leaves patients unable to put or place their hand in space effectively, because of the reduction in the arc of pronation or supination.[1,30,31]

If DRUJ instability has been identified at the time of ORIF of a distal radius fracture, and a direct repair of an injured TFC has been performed, then postoperative immobilization of the forearm and elbow is required until healing of the repaired TFC has been assured. Treatment consists of 2 percutaneous 0.062-in K-wires and a long-arm cast for 6 weeks. When the cast and pins are removed, initial efforts at rotation are frustrating to patients because of the stiffness caused by reactive fibrosis during the period of immobilization. This is to be expected. Serious efforts under the direction of a certified hand therapist to reconstitute rotation and translation of the radius/carpus/hand around the distal ulnar seat are initiated. Active, active-assisted, and passive range-of-motion exercises begin immediately, with interval long-arm splinting. At 8 postoperative weeks, dynamic orthoses (joint active splints) can be useful in providing continuous gentle load in pronation and supination. As patients attempt to regain supination, the medial 4 fingers of the opposite hand are placed on the dorsal ulna, and the thumb is placed on the distal radius metaphysis. As patients actively try to supinate, 4 medial fingers lift the ulna forward while the thumb pushes the radius backward. This exercise results in forearm rotation and translation at the DRUJ. Similarly, as patients try to pronate, the medial 4 fingers of the opposite hand push (lift) the distal ulnar shaft upward (dorsally) while the thumb pushes the distal radius away (volarly), generating rotation and translation at the DRUJ. The repaired deep, foveal fibers of the ligamentum subcruentum of the TFC provide a checkrein to supraphysiologic motion of the sigmoid fossa relative to the ulnar seat. Dynamic rotational orthoses cannot create physiologic translation of the fossa on the ulnar seat.

Eventually, after at least a few months of conscientious rehabilitation, patients should have regained full pronosupination. In spite of extensive rehabilitation, some patients may struggle and fail to achieve this goal. It is important for the surgeons to accept that forearm rotational stiffness is a potential complication in the management of fractures of the distal radius. This awareness should be communicated to patients during the early aftercare period. Rotational stiffness can result after closed or open treatment of distal radius fractures, with or without concomitant treatment of TFC or ulnar styloid pathology.

In any circumstance, restoration of a healthy forearm range of motion can be inhibited by contracture of the distal radioulnar joint capsule. A dorsal capsular contracture limits pronation; a volar contracture limits supination. Both may occur together. Like all other diarthrodial joints, the DRUJ articulating surfaces are covered by hyaline cartilage, which is nourished by the synovial tissue lining the joint. The entire joint is surrounded by elastic connective tissue forming a capsule and, as in any other diarthrodial joint, can be subjected to fibrosis and contracture during prolonged immobilization after trauma.

In 1993, laboratory and clinical work on the subject of posttraumatic DRUJ contracture was published.[30] The anatomy of the DRUJ capsule in fresh, frozen cadavers was critically studied, shedding insight into why posttrauma supination was so much more difficult to achieve than posttrauma pronation. With closed or open treatment of distal radius fractures, the magnitude of hemorrhage and swelling, combined with prolonged immobilization, is a clinical setup for loss of native DRUJ capsule elasticity, with resultant contracture that checkreins supination or pronation. Redundant folds of native volar DRUJ capsule make this portion of the capsule more susceptible to stiffness after reactive fibrosis has occurred. In most cases, commitment to rehabilitation by patient and therapist overcomes this inherent predisposition to volar or dorsal stiffness, but, in many cases, pronosupination efforts plateau too early, leaving the forearm relatively stiff, significantly compromising upper limb function.

On the basis of laboratory and clinical research produced by author and his colleague, Dr Thomas Graham[29], a surgical approach to the contracted DRUJ volar capsule in cases of limited supination and to the contracted dorsal DRUJ capsule limiting pronation was designed. Since the publication of this initial work, DRUJ capsulectomy has been used extensively at The Indiana Hand to Shoulder Center and has been accepted as a logical and reasonable approach to improving forearm rotation in patients who (1) have healed their distal radius reconstruction, (2) have had alignment restored at the DRUJ articular surfaces, and (3) have a TFC that is uninjured or has been reconstructed. It is critical for surgeons to recognize that if it has been technically impossible to restore perfect alignment of the sigmoid fossa and ulnar seat components of the DRUJ, then DRUJ capsulotomy should never be performed.[1,30,31] If there is step-off incongruity of the DRUJ articular surfaces or a poorly oriented sigmoid fossa tracking line for the principal axis of load bearing, then performing a DRUJ capsulectomy only exposes the joint to increased surface shear forces and predisposes the joint to painful, progressive degenerative cartilage breakdown and inflammation. The capsulectomy (whether or not dorsal or palmar) will fail. Postreduction (open or closed) malalignment of DRUJ articular anatomy is a significant contraindication to DRUJ capsulectomy, volar or dorsal.

If forearm rehabilitation plateaus with persistent stiffness, then surgical intervention should be considered. Because of the differences in anatomy between the dorsal and volar DRUJ capsules,[30] limited forearm supination is more commonly observed after distal radius fracture, treated closed or open. Functional limitation of supination can be treated surgically by radical silhouette capsulectomy of the entire volar radioulnar DRUJ capsule, proximal to the most proximal fibers of the ligamentum subcruentum (**Fig. 26**). Once performed, intra-operative manipulation of the forearm by rotation and translation should restore full supination. Similarly, limitation of forearm pronation can be surgically addressed by radical dorsal DRUJ silhouette capsulectomy proximal to the dorsal fibers of the TFC (**Fig. 27**). Manipulation of the forearm by rotation and translation into pronation restores a full arc of forearm motion. Any bony angulatory, rotational, or length malalignment at the DRUJ must be corrected

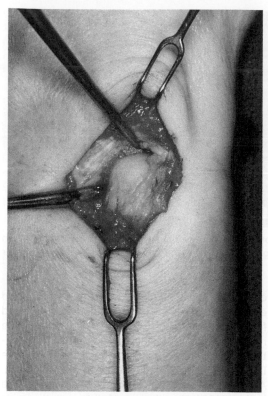

Fig. 26. Silhouette capsulectomy of the palmar DRUJ capsule must be performed proximal to the palmar ligamentum subcruentum of the TFC. The entire capsule should be removed and in any intra-articular adhesions lysed. Once this is accomplished, rotation and translation of the DRUJ should result in 90° of passive forearm supination.

before consideration can be given to DRUJ capsulectomy.

TRAUMATIC ARTHRITIS OF THE DRUJ IN ASSOCIATION WITH FRACTURE OF THE DISTAL RADIUS

Fracture extension into the DRUJ results in what is unfortunately a common complication of distal radius fractures: traumatic DRUJ arthritis. Even without comminuted fracture displacement, simple damage to the articular surface of the sigmoid fossa can result in progressive chondrolysis and exposed subchondral bone.[32] Failure to anatomically align displaced DRUJ fracture fragments can accelerate the degenerative process. **Fig. 28** shows the wrist radiographs of a 45-year-old man who incurred a high-energy industrial accident. Comminution was extensive; dorsal collapse and shortening was impressive. In spite of prolonged intraoperative efforts (with distraction) to reconstitute some semblance of

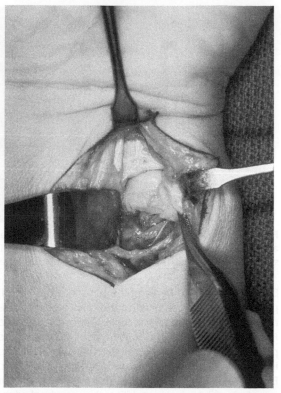

Fig. 27. Silhouette capsulectomy of the dorsal DRUJ capsule, followed by lysis of all intra-articular adhesions, should result in 90° of passive forearm pronation.

architectural alignment of joint surfaces, the result was persistent dorsal tilt at the radiocarpal joint and destruction of the DRUJ (**Fig. 29**). Predictably, the patient went on to have severe pain and stiffness with forearm rotation, requiring elimination of the DRUJ by Darrach resection of the distal ulna, stabilized by adjunctive tendon transfers (**Fig. 30**).[33]

Most surgeons today recognize the 30% reported failure rate after simple Darrach resection in the high-demand hand,[34] most commonly associated with winging or impingement of the unstable proximal stump of ulna.[35–39] Since Darrach described his procedure,[40–42] a variety of solutions have been proposed for the post-Darrach problem of proximal ulnar stump instability.[1,32]

The matched ulna resection (Watson and colleagues)[38,39] and the hemiresection interposition technique (Bowers),[36,37] popular in the 1980s, recognized the propensity for the 2 forearm bones to impinge and wing after ulnar seat-pole resection for painful DRUJ arthritis. The investigators addressed the issue by ulnar contouring with or without rolled-up tendon interposition.

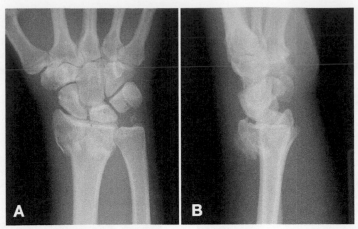

Fig. 28. (*A*) Anteroposterior and (*B*) lateral radiographs of a devastingly comminuted distal radius fracture in a 45-year-old man injured on an industrial accident. The sigmoid fossa of the radius was destroyed. The articular surface of the radiocarpal joint was severely damaged.

Synostosis of the head of the ulna to a damaged, painful sigmoid fossa, with creation of a pseudarthrosis just proximal to the fusion mass (Suavé and Kapandji),[43,44] eliminates joint pain, but subjects patients to similar problems of proximal stump instability seen with simple Darrach resection. Even Taleisnik's thoughtful use of the pronator quadratus[45] to help stabilize the proximal ulnar stump of a Sauvé-Kapandji procedure leaves patients with persistent weakness and a propensity for the ulnar stump to wing or impinge against the medial border of the radius.

During the past few decades, various attempts have been made by clinical researchers to design prostheses to replace the distal end of the ulna and provide a fulcrum for forearm rotation. These have had limited effectiveness in the higher-demand hand because of the persistent pain caused by prosthetic loading of the denuded and eburnated bone of the exposed, damaged sigmoid fossa. Scheker and coworkers[46] have made recent strides in designing a constrained prosthesis that considers both components of the DRUJ: the ulnar seat and the radius sigmoid fossa. Although the surgical technique is demanding, the logic behind the design of this prosthesis is extraordinary. Scheker and coworkers report good long-term results in their patient population.

Treatment of traumatic arthritis of the DRUJ after distal radius fracture remains a conundrum for reconstructive hand surgeons. Until a prosthesis is designed that (1) is truly user friendly, (2) is able to withstand high-demand loads, (3) makes anatomic and biomechanical sense, (4) is affordable, and (5) can be implanted technically without compromising the engineering requirements of the

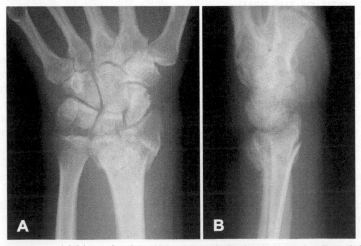

Fig. 29. (*A*) Anteroposterior and (*B*) lateral radiographs showing the healed distal radius of the patient in **Fig. 21** revealing DRUJ arthrosis and radiocarpal arthrosis. Note the severe 45° dorsal tilt of the distal radius and collapse of the lunate facet of the distal radius.

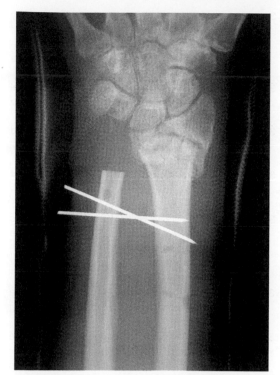

Fig. 30. Darrach resection of the distal ulna, with stump stabilization by pronator quadrates and ECU tendon transfers supplemented by convergent 0.062-in K-wires for 6 weeks, restored painless forearm rotation to the patient suffering with the DRUJ bony relationship shown in **Fig. 29**A. (*Data from* Kleinman WB, Greenberg JA. Salvage of the failed Darrach procedure. J Hand Surg Am 1995;20:951–8.)

normal DRUJ, any surgical treatment of painful DRUJ arthritis will remain challenging and frustrating to surgeons and patients alike.

This article provides insight into chronic DRUJ instability and stiffness often associated with fractures of the distal radius. Anatomic alignment and rigid fixation of distal radius fracture fragments by surgeons is only partial treatment of the injury. Surgeons must also understand and be able to focus their attention on (1) the omnipresent potential for extension of the injury into the components of the TFC, with resultant chronic DRUJ instability, and (2) contracture of the DRUJ capsule leading to stiffness of forearm rotation and thus significant compromise to global function of the upper limb.

ACKNOWLEDGMENTS

Special thanks to Gary Schnitz, my friend and colleague, who has provided all the partners of The Indiana Hand to Shoulder Center with some of the finest medical illustrations in all academic hand surgery. His brilliant work is recognized throughout the hand surgery world. His drawings have helped an untold number of students of hand surgery more clearly understand our research, our clinical work, and our professional endeavors in general.

REFERENCES

1. Kleinman WB, Graham TJ. Distal ulnar injury and dysfunction. In: Peimer CA, editor. Surgery of the hand and upper extremity. New York: McGraw-Hill; 1996. p. 667–709.
2. Kleinman WB. Stability of the distal radioulna joint: biomechanics, pathophysiology, physical diagnosis, and restoration of function what we have learned in 25 years. J Hand Surg 2007;32(7):1086–106.
3. Kleinman WB. Stability of the distal radioulnar joint. In: Slutsky DJ, Osterman AL, editors. Fractures and injuries of the distal radius and carpus. Philadelphia (PA): The Cutting Edge; 2009. p. 261–74, Chapter 25.
4. Mahmud F, Nazarian DG, Zahner EJ, et al. Creation of a "one-bone" forearm to reconstruct large radioulnar defects. Orthop Trans 1996;20(1):231.
5. Schneider LH, Imbriglia JE. Radioulnar joint fusion for distal radioulnar joint instability. Hand Clin 1991; 7(2):391–5.
6. Peterson CA 2nd, Maki S, Wood MB. Clinical results of the one-bone forearm. J Hand Surg Am 1995; 20(4):609–18.
7. Palmer AK, Glisson RR, Werner FW. Ulnar variance determination. J Hand Surg Am 1982;7(4):376–9.
8. Goldner JL, Hayes MG. Stabilization of the remaining ulna using one-half of the extensor carpi ulnaris tendon after resection of the distal ulna. Orthop Trans 1979;3:330–1.
9. Spinner M, Kaplan EB. Extensor carpi ulnaris: its relationship to stability of the distal radioulnar joint. Clin Orthop Relat Res 1970;68:124–8.
10. Ruby LK, Ferenz CC, Dell PC. The pronator quadrates interposition transfer: an adjunct to resection arthroplasty of the distal radioulnar joint. J Hand Surg Am 1996;21:60–5.
11. Hotchkiss RN, An KN, Sowa DT, et al. An anatomic and mechanical study of the interosseous membrane of the forearm: pathomechanics of the proximal migration of the radius. J Hand Surg Am 1989;14:256–61.
12. Bowers WH. Surgical procedures for the distal radioulnar joint. In: Lichtman DM, editor. The wrist and its disorders. Philadelphia: WB Saunders; 1988. p. 232–43.
13. af Ekenstam F, Hagert C. Anatomical studies on the geometry and stability of the distal radio ulnar joint. Scand J Plast Reconstr Surg 1985;19:17–25.
14. Bednar MS, Arnoczky SP, Weiland AJ. The microvasculature of the triangular fibrocartilage complex: its clinical significance. J Hand Surg Am 1991;16:1101–5.

15. Thiru-Pathi RG, Ferlic DC, Clayton ML, et al. Arterial anatomy of the triangular fibrocartilage of the wrist and its clinical significance. J Hand Surg Am 1986; 11:258–63.

16. Palmer AK, Werner FW. Biomechanics of the distal radio-ulnar joint. Clin Orthop Relat Res 1984;187:26–35.

17. Schuind F, An KN, Berglund L, et al. The distal radio-ulnar ligaments: a biomechanical study. J Hand Surg Am 1991;16:1106–14.

18. af Ekenstam FW, Palmer AK, Glisson RR. The load on the radius and ulna in different positions of the wrist and forearm: a cadaver study. Acta Orthop Scand 1984;55:363–5.

19. Kauer JM. The articular disc of the hand. Acta Anat 1975;93:590–605.

20. Hagert CG. Distal radius fracture and the distal radioulnar joint—anatomical consideration. Handchir Mikrochir Plast Chir 1994;26:22–6.

21. Palmer AK. Triangular fibrocartilage complex lesions: a classification. J Hand Surg Am 1989;14:594–606.

22. Pogue DJ, Viegas SF, Patterson RM, et al. Effects of distal radius fracture malunion on wrist joint mechanics. J Hand Surg Am 1990;15:721–7.

23. Taleisnik J, Watson HK. Midcarpal instability caused by malunited fractures of the distal radius. J Hand Surg Am 1984;9(3):350–7.

24. af Ekenstam F, Hagert CG. The distal radio ulnar joint. The influence of geometry and ligament on simulated colles' fracture. An experimental study. Scand J Plast Reconstr Surg 1985;19(1):27–31.

25. Souer JS, Ring D, Matschke S, et al. Effect of an unrepaired fracture of the ulnar styloid base on outcome after plate-and-screw fixation of a distal radial fracture. J Bone Joint Surg Am 2009;91:830–8.

26. Sammer DM, Shah HM, Shauverf MJ, et al. The effect of ulnar styloid fractures on patient-rated outcomes after volar locking plating of distal radius fractures. J Hand Surg Am 2009;34(9):1595–602.

27. Sebastiaan JS, Ring D, Matschke S, et al. Effect of an unrepaired fracture of the ulnar styloid base on outcome after plate- and screw fixation of a distal radial fracture. J Bone Joint Am 2009;91:830–8.

28. Jupiter JB. Commentary: the effect of ulnar styloid fractures on patient-rated outcomes after volar locking plating of distal radius fractures. J Hand Surg Am 2009;34(9):1603–4.

29. Hermansdorfer JD, Kleinman WB. Management of chronic peripheral tears of the triangular fibrocartilage complex. J Hand Surg Am 1991;16(2):340–6.

30. Kleinman WB, Graham TJ. The distal radioulnar joint capsule: clinical anatomy and role in posttraumatic limitation of forearm rotation. J Hand Surg Am 1998;23(4):588–99.

31. Kleinman WB. Distal radio-ulna joint capsulectomy for post-traumatic limitation of forearm rotation. In: Gelberman RH, editor. Master Techniques in Orthopaedic Surgery: The Wrist. 3rd edition. Philadelphia (PA): Lippencott; 2010. p. 411–28, Chapter 36.

32. Kleinman WB. Salvage procedures for the distal end of the ulna: there is no magic. Am J Orthop 2009;38(4):172–80.

33. Kleinman WB, Greenberg JA. Salvage of the failed Darrach procedure. J Hand Surg Am 1995;20:951–8.

34. Hartz CR, Beckenbaugh RD. Long-term results of resection of the distal ulna for post-traumatic conditions. J Trauma 1979;19(4):219–26.

35. Sauerbier M, Fujita M, Hahn ME, et al. The dynamic radio-ulnar convergence of the Darrach procedure and the ulnar head hemiresection interposition arthroplasty: a biomechanical study. J Hand Surg Br 2002;27(4):307–16.

36. Bowers WH. Distal radioulnar joint arthroplasty: the hemiresetion-interposition technique. J Hand Surg Am 1985;10(2):169–78.

37. Bowers WH. Hemiresection interposition technique (HIT) arthroplasty of the distal radioulnar joint. In: Gelberman RH, editor. The wrist: master techniques in orthopaedic surgery. New York: Raven Press; 1994. p. 303–18.

38. Watson HK, Ryu J, Burgess R. Matched distal ulnar resection. J Hand Surg Am 1986;11(6):812–7.

39. Watson HK, Gabuzda GM. Matched distal ulnar resection for posttraumatic disorders of the distal radioulnar joint. J Hand Surg Am 1992;17(4):724–30.

40. Darrach W. Forward dislocation at the inferior radioulnar joint, with fracture of the lower third of the shaft of the radius. Ann Surg 1912;56(5):801.

41. Darrach W. Anterior dislocation of the head of the ulna. Ann Surg 1912;56(5):802–3.

42. Darrach W. Partial excision of the lower shaft of ulna for deformity following Colles's fracture. Ann Surg 1913;57(5):764–5.

43. Sauvé L, Kapandji M. Nouvelle technique de traitement chirurgical des luzations récidivantes isolées de l'extrémité inferieure du cubitus [A new technique for the surgical treatment of isolated recurrent dislocations of the distal end of the ulnar]. J Chirurg 1936;47(4):589–94 [in French].

44. Kapandji AL. The Sauvé-Kapandji procedure. J Hand Surg Br 1992;17(2):125–6.

45. Taleisnik J. The Sauvé-Kapandji procedure. Clin Orthop 1992;275:110–23.

46. Scheker LR, Babb BA, Killion PE. Distal ulnar prosthetic replacement. Orthop Clin North Am 2001; 32(2):365–76.

Postoperative Infections: Prevention and Management

R. Glenn Gaston, MD[a,b],*, Marshall A. Kuremsky, MD[c]

KEYWORDS

- Postoperative • Infection • Hand • Osteomyelitis • Wrist

More than 290,000 surgical site infections (SSIs) are reported annually in the United States according to recent reports from the Centers for Disease Control and Prevention (CDC). Annual direct and indirect cost estimates as a result of SSIs are in excess of $1 billion and $10 billion, respectively. An SSI has been defined by the CDC as an infection occurring within 30 days of an operative procedure or within 1 year in the event of material implantation.[1] These infections can be further classified as either superficial (confined to the skin and subcutaneous tissues around the incision) or deep (involving the fascia, muscle, bone, or implant). The most common causative organism involved with SSIs parallels that found in normal skin flora and is *Staphylococcus aureus*. A recent epidemiologic study[2] reported that in adults, 50% to 80% of SSI isolates are pure *S aureus*, with 12% mixed flora. Gram-negative organisms are more common in immunocompromised hosts such as people with diabetes and intravenous drug abusers.

Recently there has been an alarming and increasing trend toward methicillin-resistant *S aureus* (MRSA) isolates in SSIs. In a review of 761 patients in a 3-year period from 2001 to 2003,[3] the incidence of community-acquired MRSA in hand infections nearly doubled from 34% to 61%. The incidence of MRSA has risen so dramatically that some investigators have implied that all patients presenting with hand infections should be empirically treated for MRSA.[4]

The hand is resistant to the development of infection compared with the rest of the human body; however, its uniquely intricate and confined anatomy renders it prone to significant impairment as a result of even seemingly trivial infections. SSI rates in elective hand surgery are reported to be less than 1.4%, with deep infections less than 0.3%.[5] Unlike other infections elsewhere in the body, hand infections occur frequently in the absence of fever or increased laboratory markers of infection. A recent study found that more than 75% of patients with active hand infections were afebrile and without increased C-reactive protein (CRP) and only 50% had an increased erythrocyte sedimentation rate (ESR).[2] Clinical examination therefore is of paramount importance in the diagnosis of hand infections. Delays in treatment of hand infections in particular can have devastating consequences because of the proximity of nearby critical anatomic structures to which local infection can easily spread. Dense vascular and lymph anastomoses, tendon sheaths, and deep palmar spaces all provide easy access for rapid spread of infection.

To minimize the morbidity of SSIs one must focus on modification of preoperative, intraoperative, and postoperative risk factors. If despite these efforts an SSI occurs, prompt diagnosis and management are critical. This article focuses first on the prevention of SSI through modifiable preoperative, intraoperative, and postoperative factors and second on managing established postoperative infections.

The authors have no financial disclosures or funding related to this manuscript to report.
a Carolinas Medical Center, 1000 Blythe Boulevard Charlotte, NC 28203, USA
b OrthoCarolina, 1915 Randolph Road, Charlotte, NC 28207, USA
c Department of Orthopedics, Carolinas Medical Center, Charlotte, NC 28203, USA
* Corresponding author. OrthoCarolina, 1915 Randolph Road, Charlotte, NC 28207.
E-mail address: glenngaston@hotmail.com

Hand Clin 26 (2010) 265–280
doi:10.1016/j.hcl.2010.01.002

PREOPERATIVE MODIFIABLE RISK FACTORS

Numerous modifiable preoperative risk factors have been identified and associated with increased infection risk.[6] These risk factors include malnutrition, smoking, anemia, MRSA carrier status, obesity, poor oral health, remote infection, and systemic diseases such as diabetes, human immunodeficiency virus (HIV), and rheumatoid arthritis (RA). In an elective surgical setting, many of these risk factors can be identified and optimized before surgery.

MALNUTRITION

Malnutrition is a well-recognized risk factor for deep infections in orthopedic surgery. Typically malnutrition is defined as serum albumin level less than 3.5 g/dL, total lymphocyte count less than 1500/mm^3, or a serum transferrin level less than 226 mg/dL, and wound healing complications have been associated with these levels of malnutrition. The association of malnutrition with SSI is likely multifactorial. Decreased lymphocyte counts directly decrease host cell-mediated immunity. A lack of essential vitamins and minerals such as vitamin A, vitamin C, zinc, and copper contribute indirectly toward diminished function of T lymphocytes and natural killer cells.[7,8] Furthermore, low protein levels lead to decreased angiogenesis, increased third-space fluid losses, and poor blood oxygenation.[7] In 1 study of 31 postoperative orthopedic wound complications, 27 were found to be nutritionally depleted as defined in this article.[9]

SMOKING

Smoking continues to be the leading cause of preventable morbidity and mortality in the United States. Despite the well-known risks incurred with cigarette use, there are still more than 50 million smokers consuming in excess of 800 billion cigarettes annually in the United States.[10] By virtue of its vasoconstrictive effects and tissue-induced hypoxia, smoking can also increase risk of complications with wound healing also. The tissue-induced hypoxia from smoking is caused by the binding of carbon monoxide to hemoglobin, forming carboxyhemoglobin, which deprives local tissue of available oxygen. A randomized study has shown that smoking cessation even as little as 4 to 6 weeks preoperatively can decrease postoperative complications, including with wound healing.[11]

MRSA CARRIER

S aureus is the most common organism found in 33Is, and Staphylococcus epidermidis is often associated with infections involving implants. The incidence of community-acquired MRSA in hand infections has been steadily rising in the United States.[12] The most common strain of community-acquired MRSA, termed USA 300 by the CDC, has a unique membrane toxin named Panton-Valentine leukocidin that targets host leukocytes, resulting in often severe skin infections and antibiotic resistance.[13,14]

Nasal carriage of S aureus has been associated with 2 to 9 times increased risk of SSIs.[15] Preoperative nasal swabs for Staphylococcus and specifically MRSA have recently been developed with decolonization protocols consisting of mupirocin or Bactroban ointment applied twice daily to the nares. The authors have begun using this preoperative screening protocol on all patients with major arthroplasty, including elbow and wrist arthroplasty. If swabs are positive, vancomycin is our preoperative antibiotic of choice on the day of surgery.

DIABETES

Given population prevalence estimates of nearly 10% in the United States in adults more than 50 years old, diabetes mellitus warrants special consideration.[16] Between 5% and 35% of patients requiring hospital admission for hand infections have diabetes.[17–20] A study by Mandell[21] found that 8 of 15 presumed nondiabetic patients who had recently resolved hand infections tested positive to a glucose tolerance test, suggesting a potentially high incidence of undiagnosed diabetes in this patient population.

Diabetes has been shown to affect host cell-mediated immunity, neutrophil and lymphocyte function, and wound healing.[22] However, high levels of hyperglycemia (>250 mg/dL) and metabolic acidosis are required to produce these cellular changes.[23,24] Many potentially confounding variables such as patient age, obesity, malnutrition, local tissue hypoxia caused by poor circulation, and peripheral neuropathy likely contribute also to the high association of diabetic patients with wound healing complications, including SSI. Some studies have attempted to eliminate these confounding variables using multivariate regression analysis and have found diabetes is not an independent risk factor for the development of an SSI.[25,26] Other studies have documented higher rates of SSI in patients with diabetes even after only minor soft-tissue procedures.[27,28] Evidence is now emerging from the cardiothoracic literature that tight perioperative glycemic control directly leads to a decreased incidence of SSI and mortality.[29–31]

Patients with diabetes mellitus are not only potentially more prone to developing infections but also have a higher morbidity and mortality associated with the development of infection. In the presence of an upper-extremity infection, patients with diabetes can have amputation rates up to 63% and a mortality of 19%.[32,33] In the subset of patients with diabetes with renal failure, even higher morbidity and mortality exist, with 1 study reporting an amputation rate of 100% in this cohort.[33] In the setting of infection in a patient with diabetes, early and aggressive treatment is necessary as the severity and extent of infection are frequently underestimated in this patient population.[20] Incisions should extend along the entire length of indurated or erythematous skin.

Although *S aureus* remains the most common offending pathogen, fungal, polymicrobial, and gram-negative organisms (73% in some studies) have a higher prevalence in patients with diabetes.[34] Cultures for atypical mycobacterium, fungal, and anaerobic organisms are recommended in diabetic infection, and empiric antibiotic therapy needs to be broad-spectrum.

During the perioperative period, attempts to maintain serum glucose levels between 100 and 180 mg/dL should be made to optimize the immune status and wound healing potential of patients with diabetes.

HIV

HIV suppresses the formation of CD4 T-helper cells that control cell-mediated immunity. Progressive decline in CD4 cells directly correlates with the severity of the immunocompromised state and susceptibility to infection. Much like patients with diabetes, HIV-positive patients have higher morbidity associated with infections, especially in the presence of AIDS. Although the clinical presentation is similar to non-HIV-positive patients, the course of the infection tends to be unusually aggressive. Glickel[35] termed this finding as "atypical manifestations of infection with typical organisms." In Glickel's series, 7 of 8 patients had opportunistic infections elsewhere (predominantly pneumonia), whereas none had opportunistic infections of the hand.

This aggressive nature of hand infections in HIV-positive patients becomes evident considering the reoperation rate for infection has been reported to be 29% and amputation rate 12%.[36] The high rate of intravenous drug abuse in patients with HIV is an independent risk factor for the development of infection, particularly more severe or atypical infections. Herpetic viral infections are also more common in HIV-positive patients and are more virulent in this population, with a predilection for superinfection. Necrotizing

fasciitis is more frequent in this population also, with an incidence of more than 20% in 1 recent study, although intravenous drug abuse is a confounding variable. Wound healing has not been found to be impaired in patients with HIV.[37,38] Hand surgeons should be cognizant also that in more than half of the reported cases, hand infection preceded the diagnosis of HIV in 1 series; therefore a high index of suspicion is necessary in such circumstances.[35]

RA

RA is an inflammatory arthropathy that affects 1% of the population.[39] There is a predilection for hand and upper-extremity involvement in RA, and SSI has a well-known association with RA surgery. In the literature for hip and knee arthroplasty, a two- to threefold increased risk of an SSI and 5 times higher rates of wound dehiscence have been reported for patients with RA compared with patients with osteoarthritis.[40] Similarly, elbow arthroplasty SSI rates are higher in patients with RA, with an incidence of 7% to 9%.[41,42] The increased rate of SSI in patients with RA has been believed to be due in part to the immunosuppressive effects of the disease, the immunosuppressive effects of the medications used to treat the disease, patient malnutrition, and other comorbidities.

Medications often used in the management of RA that have been implicated as possible causes of SSI include steroids, methotrexate, and tumor necrosis factor α (TNF-α) antagonists. Steroids, such as prednisone, are commonly used in the management of RA and suppress antibody formation and phagocyte function, thereby increasing susceptibility to infection.[43] Chronic steroid administration in animal models has caused delays in skin and bone healing.[44,45] Clinical studies looking at the association of long-term steroid use and wound healing complications have conflicting reports, with some studies finding an association[46,47] and others finding no association.[48,49]

Methotrexate usage during the perioperative period has been the source of much debate.[50] Concern stems from its immunosuppressive effects and impairment in wound healing in animal studies.[51,52] In addition, some clinical studies support methotrexate cessation before surgery.[53,54] Other clinical studies have found no increased risk of complications with wound healing or SSI in patients continuing methotrexate therapy throughout the perioperative period and a decreased incidence of disease flare-ups.[46,48,49,55]

Only 2 studies have looked specifically at SSI and wound healing complications in patients with

RA undergoing hand surgery on methotrexate or steroids and neither found an increased rate of complications associated with continued use of these medications throughout the perioperative period.[49,55]

A newer class of medication, TNF-α inhibitors, has recently been gaining popularity in the management of autoimmune disorders, including RA. TNF-α antagonists block the cytokine-mediated inflammatory cascade that is overexpressed in RA patients. Presently there are 3 approved TNF-α antagonists on the market: etanercept (Enbrel), infliximab (Remicade), and adalimumab (Humira). All 3 of these medications have shown superior efficacy to that of methotrexate in preventing the bone and cartilage destruction of RA.[56] Although no specific studies have investigated hand or upper-extremity infections in patients on these medications, serious infections have been seen in up to 18% of patients with RA who are receiving TNF-αtherapy.[57]

Comorbidities such as malnutrition have also been implicated in the increased prevalence of SSI and poor wound healing in patients with RA. Rayan and colleagues[58] found that malnutrition coexisted with RA in up to 75% of patients, based on serum albumin level, total lymphocyte count, triceps skin fold measurement, and midarm muscle circumference.

MASTECTOMY

Patients having previously undergone ipsilateral mastectomy with lymph node dissection were traditionally believed to have increased risk of developing an SSI as a result of localized immune impairment[59,60]; however, there is a growing body of evidence to the contrary. Hershko and Stahl[61] recently reviewed 25 cases of elective hand surgery in patients with a history of ipsilateral mastectomy with axillary lymph node dissection and found no infections or new cases of lymphedema. Similarly, 2 separate studies investigating carpal tunnel release in this patient population found no infections in a combined total of 67 cases.[62,63] Based on the available studies, this subset of patients does not seem to be at increased risk of developing an SSI; however, given the gravity of an infection in such a limb, early and aggressive treatment of any suspected cellulitis is justified.

PROPHYLACTIC ANTIBIOTICS

Many prospective, randomized trials have reported reduced rates of SSI with the use of preoperative antibiotics in patients undergoing surgery for long-bone trauma, hip fractures, and total joint arthroplasty.[64–66] In these patients a first-generation cephalosporin such as cefazolin is the antibiotic of choice in the absence of documented β-lactam allergy or known MRSA carrier status, in which case vancomycin is recommended. For cases in which β-lactam allergy is in question, skin testing for penicillin allergy is available.[67] Optimal timing of antibiotic administration is within 60 minutes of incision to ensure adequate tissue levels are present at the commencement of surgery. Studies looking at cefazolin concentration in bone at the time of incision have found levels more than 60 times the minimal inhibitory concentration.[68] No benefit has been shown in continuing prophylactic antibiotics beyond 24 hours postoperatively in preventing SSI, and it may propagate antimicrobial resistance.[69,70]

Unlike the general orthopedic literature, the role of prophylactic antibiotics in elective hand surgery is less clear, due in part to the overall extremely low infection rate of elective hand procedures. In a report of 2337 elective upper-extremity cases Kleinert and coleagues[5] found a deep infection rate of only 0.3%. Similarly, in a report of 3620 elective carpal tunnel releases, of which 80% were performed without antibiotic administration, Hanssen and colleagues[71] found an infection rate of 0.47%. A recent prospective, randomized, double-blind, placebo-controlled study by Whittaker and colleagues[72] found no difference in the rate of infection in clean, incised hand injuries with or without the use of preoperative antibiotics.

The literature does, however, have some evidence supporting the use of prophylactic antibiotics in specific elective hand procedures based on the length of procedure, specific host factors, presence of certain implants, and degree of wound contamination.[73] Procedures lasting more than 2 hours have been shown to have significantly increased risk of developing an SSI. Haley and colleagues[74] reviewed more than 58,000 surgical cases and found operative time of more than 2 hours to be an independent predictor of wound infection. Two additional studies provide level 1 evidence supporting the use of preoperative antibiotics in elective cases lasting more than 2 hours to minimize the risk of SSI.[75,76] It is therefore recommended that prophylactic antibiotics be given in all cases estimated to be of longer than 2 hours' duration.

The authors have recently synthesized all of the pertinent literature on antibiotic use for elective hand procedures and developed an algorithm through the quality-improvement program at our institution, which we are presently implementing. This algorithm is presented in **Fig. 1** and contains

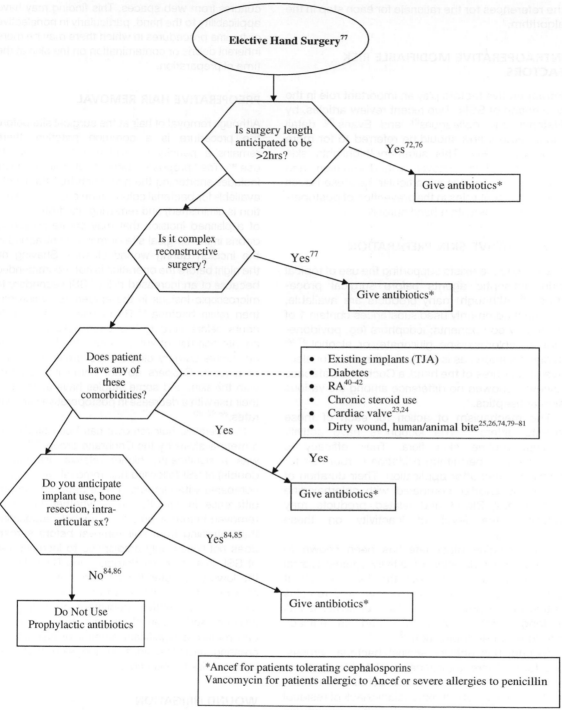

Fig. 1. Algorithm for preoperative antibiotic use. *Data from* Refs.[11,23–26,38,40–42,72,77–86]

the references for the rationale for each step in the algorithm.

INTRAOPERATIVE MODIFIABLE RISK FACTORS

Intraoperative factors play an important role in the prevention of SSIs. Two recent review articles, by Fletcher and colleagues[87] and Evans,[88] detail these factors and should be referred to for more in-depth review. This summary highlights skin preparation, hair removal, wound irrigation, and postoperative drains in particular, as these issues play prominent roles in the prevention of postoperative infections within hand surgery.

PREOPERATIVE SKIN PREPARATION

Clear evidence exists supporting the use of topical skin antiseptic agents before surgical procedures.[88] Although many products are available, the most commonly used substances contain 1 of 3 primary components: iodophors (eg, povidone-iodine), chlorhexidine gluconate, or alcohol.[87,89] In clean surgery, as is frequently the case for elective procedures of the hand, a Cochrane Database review[90] showed no difference among the various skin antiseptics.

The mechanism of action for each of these agents differs.[24] The iodophors have activity against routine skin flora. Their efficacy is enhanced by permitting oxidation in room air for a few minutes after application. Their duration of activity is shorter compared with chlorhexidine gluconate.[91] Blood and related products may impart some level of inactivity on these compounds.

Chlorhexidine gluconate has been shown to have a longer duration of activity against typical skin flora compared with the iodophors.[87] It destroys bacterial cell membranes and remains active in the presence of blood proteins. It has a long duration of activity and its efficacy continues after application.[92]

Alcohol has activity against bacteria, viruses, and fungi. There are concerns related to the flammability of this substance as it pertains to patient and surgeon safety. It has a relative lack of residual activity also, which may be relevant in procedures of longer duration. There is a 95% immediate reduction in skin flora on application; this can be increased to 99% if the applications are repeated.[93]

In a quantitative assessment of skin contamination on feet, Keblish and colleagues[94] found that use of a brush, compared with a standard applicator, was more efficacious in reducing positive cultures from web spaces. This finding may have applicability to the hand, particularly in nonelective or trauma procedures in which there may be more inherent debris or contamination on the skin at the time of preparation.

PREOPERATIVE HAIR REMOVAL

Although removal of hair at the surgical site before the procedure is a common practice, there remains a paucity of evidence to support its use.[87] The proposed benefit of hair removal includes shortening the hair (such that the length available for bacterial colonization and contamination is diminished) and removing hair from an area of a planned incision that may create additional debris in the surgical site or may be entrapped in the incision during wound closure. Shaving on the night before the operation is not recommended because of an increased risk of SSI secondary to microscopic lesions in the epidermis, which can then retain bacteria.[95] Razor use more than 24 hours before surgery has been associated with an infection risk of 20%.[96] When the hair is to be cut before surgery clippers are preferred to use of a razor. Clippers do not come into contact with the skin, and some studies have associated their use with a decrease in postoperative infection rates.[88,97–99]

Preoperative hair removal has been studied in a meta-analysis by the Cochrane group.[100] There was a significantly higher relative risk (nearly double) of SSI following hair removal with a razor compared with clippers. These data revealed no difference in infection rate whether hair was removed before a procedure or not, suggesting that refraining from hair removal before surgery does not necessarily predispose to increase risk of SSI. In a study by Seropian and Reynolds,[101] the lowest SSI rates (0.6%) were noted with use of a depilatory agent or with no hair removal at all. As an alternative, depilatory products may also be used in lieu of clippers; these products can remove a significant amount of hair without creating microabrasions in the skin that may increase risk for infection.

WOUND IRRIGATION

The use of intraoperative wound irrigation in clean surgery is another technique that may minimize SSIs.[87] In a study of patients undergoing spine surgery, there is a significant difference in the infection rate in patients who underwent wound irrigation with a povidone-iodine (0.5% infection rate) irrigant compared with those who did not (2.9%).[102] The addition of antibiotics to the irrigant solution has been common historically, although this practice is not clearly justified in the literature.[103] Significant debate continues as to whether pulsatile lavage versus bulb syringe has greater efficacy, particularly in dirty or contaminated wounds.[88] Pulsatile lavage may offer benefits in being able to deliver higher-pressure irrigation, which may be useful when debris are impacted into the soft tissue or are not grossly apparent during debridement; alternatively some investigators believe that high-pressure lavage may cause deeper penetration of bacteria within tissues, preventing its removal.[104] High-pressure pulsatile lavage may also damage bone, and thus theoretically impair healing also.[88] Other investigators have shown that high-pressure lavage can result in deep seeding of the bone or medullary canal itself.[105,106]

There is some evidence for the use of detergents, such as castile soap or benzalkonium chloride, in wound irrigation fluid. The unique feature of detergents is their ability to disrupt the forces (electrostatic and hydrophobic) that otherwise bind bacteria to human tissue.[88] In a prospective, randomized study by Anglen,[107] more than 400 open fractures of the lower extremity were irrigated with either bacitracin or castile soap. In this study, there was no difference in rates of SSI or bone healing between the 2 groups, but there was more than a twofold difference in rate of wound healing for those open fractures irrigated with bacitracin compared with castile soap.

DRAINS

Wound closure over a drain has not been proven to lower SSI rates.[87,88] Much of the literature investigating this topic has been performed in joint arthroplasty. In a study by Beer and colleagues,[108] no difference in drainage, infection, or swelling was noted in patients with bilateral knee arthroplasties with and without drains. Furthermore, a meta-analysis by Parker and colleagues[109] of more than 3600 arthroplasty wounds showed no major benefit to use of a drain in hip or knee replacement surgery, but did show a higher need for transfusion with use of a drain.

Closed suction drains are associated with less retrograde bacterial migration compared with simple conduit drains.[110] Studies have shown that wound infections are associated with contaminated drain tips; however, negative culture of drain tips is not commonly associated with surgical wound infection.[111] There does seem to be a time-dependent phenomenon associated with duration of indwelling drains and wound infection; multiple studies have shown that drains left in wounds for more than 24 hours have a higher association with wound infections.[112,113]

MANAGEMENT OF SSIs

Despite all our efforts to prevent SSI, postoperative infections will continue to occur. Although there are important general principles to follow in dealing with SSI, the treatment plan must be individualized. The first step in the management of a potential SSI is to obtain a thorough history and physical examination. The timeline for onset of symptoms should be ascertained, as earlier detection has a higher likelihood of successful management with proper immobilization and oral antibiotics alone. Also, the rapidity of symptom progression is critical, especially when considering aggressive rapidly progressing infections such as necrotizing fasciitis. The presence of hardware and stability of the underlying fracture when present must be considered. The host risk factors outlined earlier must be considered and included in the decision for potentially more aggressive management. In posttraumatic cases, the nature of the injury, especially as it relates to possible sources of infection, must be sought (eg, bite wound, soil contamination, marine environment) to help guide empiric antibiotic selection.

Physical examination should focus first on differentiating a superficial from a deep infection. The most common superficial infection is cellulitis, which manifests as erythema, warmth, swelling, tenderness, and at times loss of motion. Cellulitis can progress along lymphatic tracks, causing an ascending lymphangitis, which appears as red streaking up the arm. Regional lymphadenopathy and tenderness should be assessed about the medial epicondyle and axilla. Particular attention should be paid to assess for any areas of fluctuance, induration, or subcutaneous crepitation to suggest an underlying abscess or fasciitis, which would require prompt surgical decompression. Minor cellulitis can most often be managed with oral antibiotics such as Keflex or clindamycin (for penicillin allergy) to provide coverage for the 2 most common organisms, Streptococcus and Staphylococcus. For suspected MRSA, the only currently approved oral antibiotic by the Food and Drug Administration is linezolid; however, several studies have reported success with trimethoprim-sulfamethoxazole (Bactrim). Linezolid (Zyvox) is a new class of antibiotic known as oxazolidinone, designed specifically for MRSA and vancomycin-resistant Enterococcus faecium. It has been shown to have excellent penetration of bone and soft tissue, with nearly 100%

bioavailability by mouth. Despite these excellent antimicrobial properties, the authors reserve the use of Zyvox for only the most extreme cases because of its high cost. When considering oral treatment for suspected or culture-positive MRSA, we typically favor Bactrim DS (2 tablets twice daily).

In postoperative infection suspected to be confined to the subcutaneous tissue, initial management with immobilization, elevation, and antibiotics is appropriate. Progress should be monitored closely and if improvement is not seen in 24 to 48 hours the patient should be reassessed for possible deep-space infection or the need for intravenous antibiotics.

Advanced imaging studies in the acute postoperative infection are rarely necessary, but in more indolent presentations can be useful. Advanced imaging can also be of benefit in distinguishing superficial infections from deeper infections when the physical diagnosis is in question. Ultrasound can help identify deeper fluid collections and guide aspiration. MRI can be of great benefit, particularly in the absence of metallic hardware, in determining deep tissue involvement such as deep abscess or osteomyelitis.

If deep infection is suspected on examination or by imaging studies, surgical drainage is necessary. Cultures should be obtained at the time of debridement and antibiotic therapy tailored to the organism and extent of infection present. Antibiotic therapy should be delayed until after cultures are obtained if possible to improve culture sensitivity. If suspicion is high for an atypical organism (eg, marine environment, immunocompromised host) special media and agar plating may be necessary and the laboratory should be alerted in advance of culture delivery to increase likelihood of culture-positive results.

When surgical drainage is deemed to be necessary, careful planning of incisions is needed to avoid possible exposed hardware, tendons, or nerves. Often this is dictated by the original incision in the acute postoperative period following an open procedure, but for percutaneous surgeries or more remote SSIs more latitude exists. When possible in the digits the authors prefer midlateral incisions along the nonborder surface of the finger. In keeping with general orthopedic principles, a thorough debridement is necessary of all nonviable tissue. Wounds are then typically left open to heal by secondary intention or only loosely closed over vital structures, with drains kept in place. For larger open wounds in the hand and forearm the wound vacuum-assisted closure (VAC, Kinetic Concept Inc, San Antonio, TX, USA) has proved useful.[114]

WOUND VAC

In situations in which primary wound closure is either not possible or not desired (in favor of delayed primary closure or healing by secondary intention), the authors have found the VAC an invaluable resource. The VAC is contraindicated in the presence of untreated osteomyelitis or malignancy. The concept of the VAC was first introduced in 1997 and involves the placement of a reticulated polyurethane sponge covered with an airtight occlusive dressing and connected to a suction canister by tubing.[115] Negative pressure can then be applied. The dressing is typically changed every 2 to 3 days at the bedside unless additional operative debridement is necessary.

When applied in the setting of an SSI, the principles of thorough wound debridement must be adhered to before VAC application. Once the wound has been meticulously debrided, vital structures such as nerves and tendons should be covered with local tissue or muscle to avoid desiccation and vessels covered with local tissue or muscle to avoid hemorrhage. Catastrophic hemorrhage has been reported when the VAC was applied in contact with vessels.[116]

The negative pressure exerted on the wound has been shown to remove edema and hemorrhage, improve local circulation, and enhance granulation tissue formation. Animal studies using laser Doppler have confirmed improved local circulation by decreasing capillary afterload.[115,117–119] This improved local perfusion leads directly to improved formation of granulation tissue. Studies comparing the VAC with traditional wet-to-dry dressings have found an 80% improvement in formation of granulation tissue.[120] Despite the theory that the VAC could remove accumulating purulence, studies have failed to report reduced bacterial loads but have reported improved wound healing from significant decreases in wound surface area.[119,121] The cost of VAC therapy is nearly identical to wet-to-dry dressings when accounting for nursing personnel dressing changes ($103 per day for VAC vs $100 per day for wet-to-dry dressings).[122]

Three specific postoperative infections deserve special consideration because of the high morbidity associated with their development and will be addressed individually: septic arthritis, osteomyelitis, and necrotizing fasciitis.

SEPTIC ARTHRITIS

Septic arthritis of the hand and wrist typically results from direct inoculation but may also arise from bactericidal or adjacent spread of a deep-space infection. Although it has received little attention in the literature, this can be a vexing complication for the patient and surgeon. Classically patients with septic arthritis present with painful swelling of the involved joint, loss of motion, and significant pain with passive motion. The joint classically postures to maximize capsular distension, which in the fingers is in a slightly flexed position. Because standard laboratory markers of infection are of less value in determining the presence of infection in the hand, aspiration should be obtained if clinical suspicion is present. Aspirate should be sent for glucose level, cell count, Gram stain, and culture to look for septic arthritis and crystal analysis to rule out gout. Septic arthritis should be suspected in cases of white blood cell (WBC) count greater than 50,000 with greater than 75% polymorphonuclear lymphocytes and a glucose concentration of 40 mg less than fasting glucose level.[123,124]

Management of septic arthritis is typically prompt surgical debridement of the involved joint to prevent articular cartilage degeneration, as outcomes have been closely tied to timing of intervention.[123] Patients presenting at more than 10 days have been shown to have universally poor results.[125] Articular cartilage degeneration and even bony erosions can occur if treatment is delayed because of continued joint exudate build-up, causing rising intra-articular pressure, which impedes synovial blood supply. Furthermore, bacterial toxins and proteolytic enzymes directly degrade articular cartilage.[123]

If patients present early (<24 hours from symptom onset), initial management with intravenous antibiotics, immobilization, and elevation is appropriate with close observation. Empiric antibiotics should again target *Staphylococcus* and *Streptococcus* species, as these are the most common pathogens. In the event of symptom progression or lack of significant improvement over the first 24 to 48 hours the patient should undergo operative exploration and drainage. Should surgery be necessary, preoperative planning of incisions to avoid resultant exposed joint, tendons, or neurovascular structures is critical.

In the wrist, a midline dorsal incision is used followed by arthrotomy between the third and fourth compartments. A recent trend toward arthroscopic debridement of septic arthritis of the wrist has developed, with results reported superior to open techniques with respect to length of hospital stay and need for repeat surgeries.[126]

For the metacarpophalangeal joints of the hand, the authors prefer a dorsal incision and then accessing the joint with an extensor splitting approach although often a traumatic arthrotomy is present through which the joint can be accessed. Release of the proximal aspect of the sagittal band fibers is also an appropriate method.

For the interphalangeal joints of the hand, we prefer a midlateral approach to access the joint either between the extensor mechanism and proper collateral ligament or between the accessory collateral ligament and volar plate. Avoiding the extensor mechanism at this level can help minimize the risk of iatrogenic swan neck or boutonniere deformity. Care must be taken, however, to avoid injury to the neurovascular bundle, which can be displaced as a result of significant digital swelling.

The skin is always left open to heal by secondary intention or closed loosely over a drain with the hand and wrist splinted in a position of function and elevated. Intravenous antibiotics are continued until systemic and local signs of infection have resolved, then a transition to oral antibiotics based on culture results for an additional 2 to 4 weeks is warranted.[124] Early hand therapy (preferably within 2 days) should be instituted as loss of motion is a significant problem, especially in the early postoperative period.[127]

OSTEOMYELITIS

By definition osteomyelitis is an infection involving bone. Osteomyelitis of the hand and wrist is rare compared with other locations in the body, accounting for less than 10% of reported cases. Postoperative osteomyelitis has been reported in 0% to 2.5% of hand cases following internal fixation of fractures.[128,129] Osteomyelitis can also result from direct extension of septic arthritis or deep abscess into bone and in rare cases by hematogenous spread or pin-track infection. Again *Staphylococcus* and *Streptococccus* are the most common organisms.

Presentation can be more subtle than other hand infections but include local erythema, swelling, warmth, tenderness, loss of motion, and at times a draining sinus. Systemic symptoms are rare. Although most patients will have local signs of inflammation, it has been reported that only one-third may have fever or increased WBC counts.[130] In cases of acute osteomyelitis, radiographs are typically negative, with the earliest radiographic sign being swelling of the soft tissue. Two or 3 weeks later, osteopenia, sclerosis, and periosteal reactions may be seen. In chronic cases, sequestrum (focus of necrotic bone) and involucrum may be seen. Many advanced imaging modalities have been used to diagnose osteomyelitis. Overall, the sensitivity and specificity of these tests is lower than might be expected for peripheral, chronic cases of osteomyelitis (**Table 1**).[131] Bone biopsy and culture remain the gold standard for diagnosis.

Although in some cases acute osteomyelitis may be effectively managed with antibiotics alone before sequestrum formation, most cases are best managed with a combined surgical and medical treatment. Surgery should be approached similar to a tumor case with an emphasis on adequate thorough debridement of all nonviable tissue. A salvage protocol must then encompass systemic or local antibiotics, skeletal stability, soft-tissue coverage, and bone grafting.[132] A complete review of this reconstructive ladder is beyond the scope of this article but a review by Zalavras and colleagues[132] should be referred to. In cases of retained hardware, stability of the bone and hardware must be assessed. If the fracture is healed and stable, the hardware should be removed. If the implant is loose, it should be removed and external fixation applied if the bone is unstable. If hardware is well fixed, an individualized approach must be used with either hardware retention with suppressive antibiotics until fracture union or hardware removal, external fixation, and possible late hardware replacement. When possible, hardware removal is favored because of the protective barrier known as biofilm associated with implants that renders antibiotic therapy less effective.

In patients in whom segments of bone require removal, cement spacers impregnated with an antibiotic can be a useful adjunct to maintain bone and soft-tissue length and provide local antibiotic delivery. Late reconstruction is then planned based on the size of the structural defect, with most cases involving less than 6-cm defects being amenable to autogenous iliac crest bone grafts and cases greater than 6 cm often necessitating vascularized grafts such as free fibula transfer (**Figs. 2** and **3**).

Prolonged intravenous antibiotics are frequently required for a 4- to 6-week minimum based on the severity of the infection and virulence of the organism. ESR and CRP levels can be helpful to follow eradication of infection. Despite aggressive management, osteomyelitis (especially of the tubular bones of the hand) can lead to marked disability, with amputation rates approaching 40% in some studies.[133]

NECROTIZING FASCIITIS

Necrotizing fasciitis is a rapidly advancing life-threatening infection of the skin, subcutaneous tissue, and fascia. There is a predilection for involvement of the extremities and a high association with intravenous drug use (63% in 1 study).[134] Based on the bacteriology, 2 types of necrotizing fasciitis have been described. Type 1 infection is most common (80% of cases) and is caused by mixed aerobic and anaerobic bacteria, including nongroup A streptococci. Type 2 infections are caused by group A streptococci alone or in combination with *Staphylococcus* species.[135]

Initially, necrotizing fasciitis may present similar to cellulitis with erythema and swelling but typically with more intense focal pain. Pain with palpation outside the zone of cellulitis should heighten concern for possible necrotizing fasciitis. Often more extensive nonpitting edema is present beyond the zone of erythema with tense, shiny skin. As the infection spreads, the initial zone of involvement grows, assumes a darker dusky hue (often gray in appearance), bullae may begin to appear, the skin may become anesthetic, subcutaneous crepitation may rarely be palpable, complaints of pain intensify, and hemodynamic instability may ensue **Fig. 4**.[136] These infections can spread rapidly, even in a few hours, and early adequate surgical debridement is the cornerstone of treatment.

Surgical debridement must be extensive (typically far beyond the expected zone of involvement). Findings of a fibrinous, necrotic tissue with what has been called "dish-water pus" tracking along the fascial plane are diagnostic. Subcutaneous vessel thrombosis and liquefaction of subcutaneous fat is typically present also. Blunt finger dissection along the involved fascial planes

Table 1
Sensitivity and specificity of osteomyelitis tests

Test	Sensitivity (%)	Specificity (%)
Positron emission tomography scan	96	91
Bone scan	82	25
Labeled WBC scan	84	80
Magnetic resonance imaging	84	60

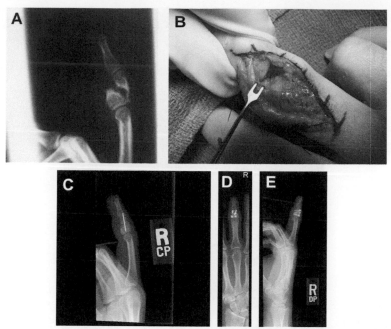

Fig. 2. (*A*) Preoperative lateral radiograph of middle phalanx osteomyelitis. (*B*) Intraoperative photograph following debridement. (*C*) Postoperative lateral with antibiotic polymethylmethacrylate (PMMA) spacer in place. (*D*) Final anteroposterior radiograph after removal of spacer and iliac crest graft placement. (*E*) Final lateral radiograph.

is easily accomplished. Wide debridement of all nonviable skin, subcutaneous fat, fascia, and at times muscle is critical, with amputation sometimes necessary. Moist dressings should then be applied and wounds left open with subsequent operative debridements every 1 to 2 days until the patient and wound have stabilized and all nonviable tissue has been excised. Multiple debridements are typically necessary and coverage with skin grafts or flaps common.

Intense medical management for fluid resuscitation and broad-spectrum intravenous antibiotics are needed. Despite aggressive management, mortality ranges from 33% to 76% even in healthy young adults, with the single most important determinant of mortality being early and adequate debridement.[134,137] Additional negative prognostic factors of outcome include age greater than 50 years, diabetes and other chronic illnesses, and involvement of the chest wall.[137]

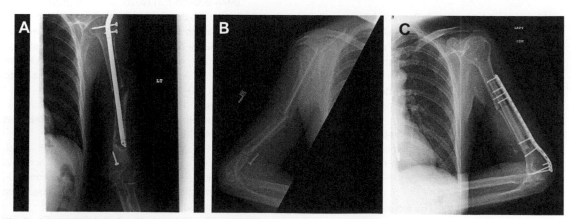

Fig. 3. (*A*) Humeral shaft osteomyelitis following intramedullary rod placement. (*B*) Postdebridement and placement of antibiotic PMMA spacer with intramedullary component. (*C*) Final radiograph following free fibula reconstruction.

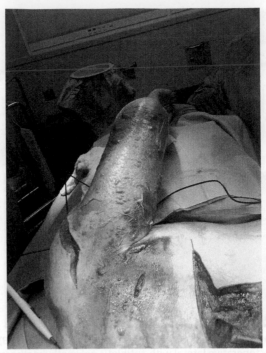

Fig. 4. Clinical photograph of necrotizing fasciitis. (*Courtesy of* Alan Ward, MD.)

SUMMARY

Postoperative infections continue to be a challenging problem. The incidence of bacterial antibiotic resistance such as MRSA is rising. There are numerous intrinsic patient factors that should be optimized before surgery to minimize the risk of SSIs. When postoperative infections develop, treatment must be individualized; however, the principles outlined in this article can help guide treatment.

REFERENCES

1. Mangrum AJ, Horan TC, Pearson ML, et al. Guideline for prevention of surgical site infection, 1999. Hospital Infection Control Practices Advisory Committee. Infect Control Hosp Epidemiol 1999; 20:250–78.
2. Houshian S, Seyedipour S, Wedderkopp N. Epidemiology of bacterial hand infections. Int J Infect Dis 2006;10(4):315–9.
3. LeBlanc DM, Reece EM, Horton JB, et al. Increasing incidence of methicillin-resistant *Staphylococcus aureus* in hand infections: a 3-year county hospital experience. Plast Reconstr Surg 2007;119(3):935–40.
4. Wilson PC, Rinker B. The incidence of methicillin-resistant *Staphylococcus aureus* in community-acquired hand infections. Ann Plast Surg 2009; 62(5):513–6.
5. Kleinert JM, Hoffman J, Miller Cran G, et al. Postoperative infection in a double-occupancy operating room. J Bone Joint Surg Am 1997;79:503–13.
6. The American Academy of Orthopedic Surgeons Patient Safety Committee, Evans RP. Surgical site infection prevention and control: an emerging paradigm. J Bone Joint Surg 2009;91(6):2–9.
7. Hansen P, Parvizi J. Links between malnutrition and infection are established. Orthopedics Today, November 19, 2009.
8. Fairfield KM, Fletcher RH. Vitamins for chronic disease prevention in adults: scientific review. JAMA 2002;287:3116–26.
9. Jensen JE, Jensen TG, Smith TK, et al. Nutrition in orthopaedic surgery. J Bone Joint Surg Am 1982; 64(9):1263–72.
10. Porter SE, Hanley EN Jr. The musculoskeletal effects of smoking. J Am Acad Orthop Surg 2001;9(1):9–17.
11. Lindgren L. Postoperative orthopaedic infections in patients with diabetes mellitus. Acta Orthop Scand 1973;44:149–51.
12. Kiran RV, McCampbell B, Angeles AP, et al. Increased prevalence of community-acquired methicillin-resistant *Staphylococcus aureus* in hand infections at an urban medical centre. Plast Reconstr Surg 2006;118:161.
13. Lina G, Piemont Y, Godail-Gamot F, et al. Involvement of Panton-Valentine leukocidin-producing *Staphylococcus aureus* in primary

skin infections and pneumonia. Clin Infect Dis 1999;29:1128–32.

14. McDougal LK, Steward CD, Killgore GE, et al. Pulsed-field gel electrophoresis typing of oxacillin-resistant *Staphylococcus* isolates from United States: establishing a national database. J Clin Microbiol 2003;41:5113–20.

15. Morange-Saussier V, Giraudeau B, Van der Mee N, et al. Nasal carriage of methicillin-resistant *Staphylococcus aureus* in vascular surgery. Ann Vasc Surg 2006;20:767–72.

16. Calvet H, Yoshikawa T. Infections in diabetes. Infect Dis Clin North Am 2001;15:407–21.

17. Stern PJ, Staneck JL, McDonough JJ, et al. Established hand infections: a controlled, prospective study. J Hand Surg 1983;8:553.

18. Glass KD. Factors related to the resolution of treated hand infections. J Hand Surg 1982;7:388.

19. Maloon S, deBeer JV, Opitz M, et al. Acute flexor tendon sheath infections. J Hand Surg 1990;15:474.

20. Gunther SF, Gunther SB. Diabetic hand infections. Hand Clin 1998;14(4):647–56.

21. Mandell MA. Hand infections and diabetes mellitus. Contemp Orthop 1979;1:25.

22. Phillips LG, Geldner P, Brou J. Correction of diabetic incisional healing impairment with basic fibroblast growth factor. Surg Forum 1990;41:602.

23. Shapiro DB. Postoperative infection in hand surgery: cause, prevention, and treatment. Hand Clin 1994;10:1–12.

24. Shapiro DB. Postoperative infection in hand surgery. Hand Clin 1998;14(4):669–81.

25. Culver DH, Horan TC, Gaynes RP, et al. Surgical wound infection rates by wound class, operative procedure, and patient risk index. National Nosocomial Infections Surveillance System. Am J Med 1991;91(Suppl 3B):152S–7S.

26. Garibaldi RA, Cushing D, Lerer T. Risk factors for post-operative infection. Am J Med 1991;91:158S–63S.

27. Gleckman R, Al-Wawi M. A review of selective infections in the adult diabetic. Compr Ther 1999;25:109–13.

28. Gonzalez MH, Bochar S, Novotny J, et al. Upper extremity infections in patients with diabetes mellitus. J Hand Surg 1999;24(4):682–6.

29. Furnary AP, Gao G, Grunkemeier GL, et al. Continuous insulin infusion reduces mortality in patients with diabetes undergoing coronary artery bypass grafting. J Thorac Cardiovasc Surg 2003;125(5):1007–21.

30. Furnary AP, Zerr KJ, Grunkemeier GL, et al. Continuous intravenous insulin infusion reduces the incidence of deep sternal wound infection in diabetic patients after cardiac surgical procedures. Ann Thorac Surg 1999;67(2):352–60.

31. Zerr KJ, Furnary AP, Grunkemeier GL, et al. Glucose control lowers the risk of wound infection in diabetics after open heart operations. Ann Thorac Surg 1997;63(2):356–61.

32. Benotmane A, Faraoun K, Mohammedi F. Infections of the upper extremity in hospitalized diabetic patients: a prospective study. Diabetes Metab 2004;30(1):91–7.

33. Francel TJ, Marshall KA, Savage RC. Hand infections in the diabetic and the diabetic renal transplant recipient. Ann Plast Surg 1990;24(4):304–9.

34. Kour AK, Looi KP, Phone MH, et al. Hand infections in patients with diabetes. Clin Orthop Relat Res 1996;331:238–44.

35. Glickel SZ. Hand infections in patients with acquired immunodeficiency syndrome. J Hand Surg 1988;13(5):770.

36. Gonzalez MH, Nikoleit J, Weinzweig N, et al. Upper extremity infections in patients with the human immunodeficiency virus. J Hand Surg Am 1998;23:348–52.

37. Buehrer JL, Weber DJ, Meyer AA, et al. Wound infection rates after invasive procedures in HIV-1 seropositive versus HIV-1 seronegative hemophiliacs. Ann Surg 1990;211:492–8.

38. Weber DJ, Becherer PR, Rutala WA, et al. Nosocomial infection rate as a function of human immunodeficiency virus type 1 status in hemophiliacs. Am J Med 1991;91(Suppl 3B):206S–12S.

39. Akil M, Amos RS. ABC of rheumatology: rheumatoid arthritis–I: clinical features and diagnosis. BMJ 1995;310:587–90.

40. White RH, McCurdy SA, Marder RA. Early morbidity after total hip arthroplasty: rheumatoid arthritis versus osteoarthritis. J Gen Intern Med 1990;5:3034.

41. Wolfe SW, Figge MP, Ingles AE, et al. Management of infection about total elbow prosthesis. J Bone Joint Surg Am 1990;72:198–212.

42. Morrey BF, Adam R, Bryan RS. Infection after total elbow arthroplasty. J Bone Joint Surg Am 1983;65:330–8.

43. National Research Council. Postoperative wound infection: the influence of ultraviolet irradiation of the operating room and various other factors. Ann Surg 1964;160(Suppl):1–192.

44. Waters RV, Gamradt SC, Asnis P, et al. Systemic corticosteroids inhibit bone healing in a rabbit ulnar osteotomy model. Acta Orthop Scand 2000;71:316–21.

45. Cross SE, Naylor IL, Coleman RA, et al. An experimental model to investigate the dynamics of wound contraction. Br J Plast Surg 1995;48:189–97.

46. Grennan DM, Gray J, Loudon J, et al. Methotrexate and early postoperative complications in patients with rheumatoid arthritis undergoing

elective orthopaedic surgery. Ann Rheum Dis 2001;60:214–7.

47. Garner RW, Mowat AG, Hazleman BL. Post-operative wound healing in patients with rheumatoid arthritis. Ann Rheum Dis 1973;32:273–4.

48. Perhala RS, Wilke WS, Clough JD, et al. Local infectious complications following large joint replacement in rheumatoid arthritis patients treated with methotrexate versus those not treated with methotrexate. Arthritis Rheum 1991;34:146–52.

49. Jain A, Witbreuk M, Ball C, et al. Influence of steroids and methotrexate on wound complications after elective hand and wrist surgery. J Hand Surg 2002;27:449–55.

50. Steuer A, Keat AC. Perioperative use of methotrexate – a survey of clinical practice in the UK. Br J Rheumatol 1997;36:1009–11.

51. Cohen SC, Gabelnick HL, Johnson RK, et al. Effects of antineoplastic agents on wound healing in mice. Surgery 1975;78:238–44.

52. Shamberger RC, Devereux DF, Brennan MF. The effect of chemotherapeutic agents on wound healing. Int Adv Surg Oncol 1981;4:15–58.

53. Bridges SL Jr, Lopez-Mendez A, Han KH, et al. Should methotrexate be discontinued before elective orthopedic surgery in patients with rheumatoid arthritis? J Rheumatol 1991;18:984–8.

54. Carpenter MT, West SG, Vogelgesang SA, et al. Postoperative joint infections in rheumatoid arthritis patients on methotrexate therapy. Orthopedics 1996;19:207–10.

55. Kasdan ML, June L. Postoperative results of rheumatoid arthritis patients on methotrexate at the time of reconstructive surgery of the hand. Orthopedics 1993;16:1233–5.

56. Donahue KE, Gartlehner G, Jonas DE, et al. Systematic review: comparative effectiveness and harms of disease modifying medications for rheumatoid arthritis. Ann Intern Med 2008;148: 124–34.

57. Kroesen S, Widmer AF, Tyndall A, et al. Serious bacterial infections in patients with rheumatoid arthritis under TNF-α therapy. Rheumatology 2003;42:617–21.

58. Rayan GM, McCormack ST, Hoelzer DJ, et al. Nutrition and the rheumatoid hand patient. J Okla State Med Assoc 1989;82:505.

59. Calkins ER. Nosocomial infections in hand surgery. Hand Clin 1998;14(4):531–45.

60. Simon MS, Cody RL. Cellulitis after lymph node dissection for carcinoma of the breast. Am J Med 1992;93:543.

61. Hershko DD, Stahl S. Safety of elective hand surgery following axillary lymph node dissection for breast cancer. Breast J 2007;13(3):287–90.

62. Dawson WJ, Elenz DR, Winchester DP, et al. Elective hand surgery in the breast cancer patient with prior ipsilateral axillary dissection. Ann Surg Oncol 1995;2(2):132–7.

63. Assmus H, Staub F. Postmastectomy lymphedema and carpal tunnel syndrome: surgical considerations and advice for patients. Handchir Mikrochir Plast Chir 2004;36(4):237–40.

64. Boyd RJ, Burke JF, Colton T. A double-blind clinical trial of prophylactic antibiotics in hip fractures. J Bone Joint Surg Am 1973;55:1251–8.

65. Gatell JM, Riba J, Lozano ML, et al. Prophylactic cefamandole in orthopedic surgery. J Bone Joint Surg Am 1984;66:1219.

66. Schulitz KP, Winkelmann W, Schoening B. The prophylactic use of antibiotics in alloarthroplasty of the hip for coxarthrosis. Arch Orthop Trauma Surg 1980;96:79–82.

67. Li JT, Markus PJ, Osmon DR, et al. Reduction of vancomycin use in orthopedic patients with a history of antibiotic allergy. Mayo Clin Proc 2000;75:902–6.

68. Cunha BA, Gossling HR, Pasternak HS, et al. The penetration characteristics of cefazolin, cephalothin, and cephradine into bone in patients undergoing total hip replacement. J Bone Joint Surg Am 1977;59:856–9.

69. Dellinger EP, Gross PA, Barrett TL, et al. Quality standard for antimicrobial prophylaxis in surgical procedures. Infectious Diseases Society of America. Clin Infect Dis 1994;18:422–7.

70. Oishi CS, Carrion WV, Hoaglund FT. Use of parenteral prophylactic antibiotics in clean orthopedic surgery. A review of the literature. Clin Orthop Relat Res 1972;296:249–55.

71. Hanssen AD, Amadio PC, DeSilva SP. Deep postoperative wound infection after carpal tunnel release. J Hand Surg Am 1989;14:869–73.

72. Whittaker JP, Nancarrow JD, Sterne GD. The role of antibiotic prophylaxis in clean incised hand injuries: a prospective randomized placebo controlled double blind trial. J Hand Surg Br 2005;30:162–7.

73. Rizvi M, Bille B, Holtom P, et al. The role of prophylactic antibiotics in elective hand surgery. J Hand Surg Am 2008;33:413–20.

74. Haley RW, Culver DH, Morgan W, et al. Identifying patients at high risk of surgical wound infection. Am J Epidemiol 1985;121:206–15.

75. Classen DC, Evans RS, Pestotnik SL, et al. The timing of prophylactic administration of antibiotics and the risk of surgical wound infection. N Engl J Med 1992;326:281–6.

76. Henley BM, Jones RE, Wyatt RWB, et al. Prophylaxis with cefamandole nafate in elective orthopedic surgery. Clin Orthop 1986;209:249–54.

77. Amland PF, Andenaes K, Smadal F, et al. A prospective, double blind, placebo controlled trial of a single dose of azithromycin on postoperative

wound infections in plastic surgery. Plast Reconstr Surg 1995;96:948–56.

78. Ehrenkranz NJ. Surgical wound infection occurrence in clean operations. Am J Med 1981;70:909–14.

79. Haley RW. Nosocomial infections in surgical patients: developing valid measures of intrinsic patient risk. Am J Med 1991;91(Suppl 3B):145S–51S.

80. Cummings P. Antibiotics to prevent infection in patients with dog bite wounds: a meta-analysis of randomized trials. Ann Emerg Med 1994;23:535–40.

81. Platt AJ, Page RE. Postoperative infection following hand surgery. J Hand Surg Br 1995;20:685–90.

82. Mishriki SF, Law DJW, Jeffrey PJ. Factors affecting the incidence of postoperative wound infection. J Hosp Infect 1990;16:223–30.

83. Swanson AB. Flexible implant arthroplasty for arthritic finger joints. Rationale, technique, and results of treatment. J Bone Joint Surg Am 1972;54:435–55.

84. Botte MJ, Davis JLW, Rose BA. Complications of smooth pin fixation of fractures and dislocations in the hand and wrist. Clin Orthop Relat Res 1992;276:194–201.

85. Furnes A, Havelin LI, Engesaeter LB, et al. [Quality control of prosthetic replacements of knee, ankle, toe, shoulder, elbow and finger joint in Norway 1994. A report after the first year of registration of joint prostheses in the national registry]. Tidsskr Nor Laegeforen 1996;116:177 [in Norwegian].

86. Swanson AB. Flexible implant arthroplasty in the proximal interphalangeal joint of the hand. J Hand Surg Am 1985;10:796–805.

87. Fletcher N, Sofianos D, Berkes MB, et al. Prevention of perioperative infection. J Bone Joint Surg Am 2007;89:1605–18.

88. Evans RP. Surgical site infection prevention and control: an emerging paradigm. J Bone Joint Surg Am 2009;91(Suppl 6):2–9.

89. Spillane CB, Dabo MN, Fletcher NC, et al. The dichotomy in the DNA-binding behaviour of ruthenium(II) complexes bearing benzoxazole and benzothiazole groups. J Inorg Biochem 2008;102:673–83.

90. Edwards PS, Lipp A, Holmes A. Preoperative skin antiseptics for preventing surgical wound infections after clean surgery. Cochrane Database Syst Rev 2004;(3):CD003949.

91. Aly R, Maibach HI. Comparative antibacterial efficacy of a 2-minute surgical scrub with chlorhexidine gluconate, povidone-iodine, and chloroxylenol sponge-brushes. Am J Infect Control 1988;16:173–7.

92. Dahl J, Wheeler B, Mukherjee D. Effect of chlorhexidine scrub on postoperative bacterial counts. Am J Surg 1990;159:486–8.

93. Ayliffe GA. Surgical scrub and skin disinfection. Infect Control 1984;5:23–7.

94. Keblish DJ, Zurakowski D, Wilson MG, et al. Preoperative skin preparation of the foot and ankle: bristles and alcohol are better. J Bone Joint Surg Am 2005;87:986–92.

95. Briggs M. Principles of closed surgical wound care. J Wound Care 1997;6:288–92.

96. Cruse PJ, Foord R. The epidemiology of wound infection. A 10-year prospective study of 62,939 wounds. Surg Clin North Am 1980;60:27–40.

97. Kaul AF, Jewett JF. Agents and techniques for disinfection of the skin. Surg Gynecol Obstet 1981;152:677–85.

98. Alexander JW, Fischer JE, Boyajian M, et al. The influence of hair-removal methods on wound infections. Arch Surg 1983;118:347–52.

99. Balthazar ER, Colt JD, Nichols RL. Preoperative hair removal: a random prospective study of shaving versus clipping. South Med J 1982;75:799–801.

100. Tanner J, Woodings D, Moncaster K. Preoperative hair removal to reduce surgical site infection. Cochrane Database Syst Rev 2006;(3):CD004122.

101. Seropian R, Reynolds BM. Wound infections after preoperative depilatory versus razor preparation. Am J Surg 1971;121:251–4.

102. Cheng MT, Chang MC, Wang ST, et al. Efficacy of dilute betadine solution irrigation in the prevention of postoperative infection of spinal surgery. Spine (Phila Pa 1976) 2005;30:1689–93.

103. Roth RM, Gleckman RA, Gantz NM, et al. Antibiotic irrigations. A plea for controlled clinical trials. Pharmacotherapy 1985;5:222–7.

104. Hassinger SM, Harding G, Wongworawat MD. High-pressure pulsatile lavage propagates bacteria into soft tissue. Clin Orthop Relat Res 2005;439:27–31.

105. Kalteis T, Lehn N, Schroder HJ, et al. Contaminant seeding in bone by different irrigation methods: an experimental study. J Orthop Trauma 2005;19:591–6.

106. Bhandari M, Adili A, Lachowski RJ. High pressure pulsatile lavage of contaminated human tibiae: an in vitro study. J Orthop Trauma 1998;12:479–84.

107. Anglen JO. Comparison of soap and antibiotic solutions for irrigation of lower-limb open fracture wounds. A prospective, randomized study. J Bone Joint Surg Am 2005;87:1415–22.

108. Beer KJ, Lombardi AV Jr, Mallory TH, et al. The efficacy of suction drains after routine total joint arthroplasty. J Bone Joint Surg Am 1991;73:584–7.

109. Parker MJ, Roberts CP, Hay D. Closed suction drainage for hip and knee arthroplasty. A meta-analysis. J Bone Joint Surg Am 2004;86:1146–52.

110. Raves JJ, Slifkin M, Diamond DL. A bacteriologic study comparing closed suction and simple conduit drainage. Am J Surg 1984;148:618–20.

111. Sankar B, Ray P, Rai J. Suction drain tip culture in orthopaedic surgery: a prospective study of 214 clean operations. Int Orthop 2004;28:311–4.

112. Drinkwater CJ, Neil MJ. Optimal timing of wound drain removal following total joint arthroplasty. J Arthroplasty 1995;10:185–9.

113. Manian FA, Meyer PL, Setzer J, et al. Surgical site infections associated with methicillin-resistant *Staphylococcus aureus*: do postoperative factors play a role? Clin Infect Dis 2003;36:863–8.

114. Prasarn ML, Zych G, Ostermann PAW. Wound management for severe open fractures: use of antibiotic bead pouches and vacuum-assisted closure. Am J Orthop 2009;38(11):559–63.

115. Morykwas MJ, Simpson J, Punger K, et al. Vacuum-assisted closure: state of basic research and physiologic foundation. Plast Reconstr Surg 2006;117(7 Suppl):121S–6S.

116. White RA, Miki RA, Kazmier P, et al. Vacuum-assisted closure complicated by erosion and hemorrhage of the anterior tibial artery. J Orthop Trauma 2005;19(1):56–9.

117. Morykwas MJ, Argenta LC, Shelton-Brown EI, et al. Vacuum-assisted closure: a new method for wound control and treatment. Animal studies and basic foundation. Ann Plast Surg 1997;38(6):553–61.

118. Xu L, Chen SZ, Qiao C. Effects of negative pressure on wound blood flow. J Fourth Milit Med Univ 2000;21:967.

119. Agenta LC, Morykwas MJ, Marks MW, et al. Vacuum-assisted closure: state of clinic art. Plast Reconstr Surg 2006;117(7 Suppl):127S–42S.

120. DeFranzo AJ, Argenta LC, Marks MW, et al. The use of vacuum-assisted closure therapy for the treatment of lower extremity wounds with exposed bone. Plast Reconstr Surg 2001;108(5):1184–91.

121. Moues CM, Vos MC, van den Bemd GJ, et al. Bacterial load in relation to vacuum-assisted closure wound therapy: a prospective randomized trial. Wound Repair Regen 2004;12(1):11–7.

122. Herscovici D, Sanders RW, Scaduto JM, et al. Vacuum-assisted wound closure therapy (VAC therapy) for the management of patients with high-energy soft tissue injuries. J Orthop Trauma 2003;17(10):683–7.

123. Freeland AE, Senter BS. Septic arthritis and osteomyelitis. Hand Clin 1989;5:533–52.

124. Abrams RA, Botte MJ. Hand infections: treatment recommendations for specific types. J Am Acad Orthop Surg 1996;4(4):219–30.

125. Boustred AM, Singer M, Hudsen DA, et al. Septic arthritis of the metacarpophalangeal joint and interphalangeal joints of the hand. Ann Plast Surg 1999; 42(6):623–8.

126. Sammer DM, Shin AY. Comparison of arthroscopic and open treatment of septic arthritis of the wrist. J Bone Joint Surg Am 2009;91:1387–93.

127. Sinha M, Jain S, Woods DA. Septic arthritis of the small joints of the hand. J Hand Surg Br 2006; 31(6):665–72.

128. Chow SP, Pun WK, So YC, et al. Prospective study of 245 open distal fractures of the hand. J Hand Surg Br 1991;16:137.

129. Duncan RW, Freeland AF, Jabaley ME, et al. Open hand fractures: an analysis of the recovery of motion and complications. J Hand Surg 1993;18:387.

130. Waldvogel F, Medoff G, Swartz M. Osteomyelitis: a review of clinical features, therapeutic considerations and unusual aspects (second of three parts). N Engl J Med 1970;282:260–6.

131. Termaat MF, Raimakers PGHM, Scholten HJ, et al. The accuracy of diagnostic imaging for the assessment of chronic osteomyelitis: a systematic review and meta-analysis. J Bone Joint Surg Am 2005; 87:2464–71.

132. Zalavras CG, Marcus RE, Levin LS, et al. Management of open fractures and subsequent complications. J Bone Joint Surg Am 2007; 89(4):884–95.

133. Reilly KE, Linz JC, Stern PJ, et al. Osteomyelitis of the tubular bones of the hand. J Hand Surg Am 1997;22:644–9.

134. Schecter W, Meyer A, Schecter G, et al. Necrotizing fasciitis of the upper extremity. J Hand Surg 1982;7:15–20.

135. Giuliano A, Lewis F, Hadley K. Bacteriology of necrotizing fasciitis. Am J Surg 1977;134:52.

136. Gonzalez MH. Necrotizing fasciitis and gangrene of the upper extremity. Hand Clin 1998;14(4):635–45.

137. Wilkerson R, Paull W, Coville FV. Necrotizing fasciitis: a review of the literature and case report. Clin Orthop 1987;216:187–92.

Complex Regional Pain Syndrome After Hand Surgery

Zhongyu Li, MD, PhD, Beth P. Smith, PhD*,
Christopher Tuohy, MD, Thomas L. Smith, PhD,
L. Andrew Koman, MD

KEYWORDS

• Chronic pain • Upper extremity • Fracture

After an emergent or elective upper extremity surgery, complex regional pain syndrome (CRPS) may complicate recovery, delay return to work, diminish health-related quality of life, and increase the likelihood of poor outcomes and/or litigation. The clinical entity of CRPS is chronic pain that persists in the absence of ongoing cellular damage and is characterized by autonomic dysfunction, trophic changes, and impaired function. In the perioperative period, the physiologic consequences of CRPS in the upper extremity contribute to or create one or more of the following: clinically significant osteopenia, delayed bony healing or nonunion, joint stiffness, tendon adhesions, arthrofibrosis, pseudo-Dupuytren palmar fibrosis, swelling, and atrophy. This article discusses the diagnosis, physiology, and management of postsurgical CRPS that occurs after hand surgery.

INCIDENCE AND SIGNIFICANCE

Although the exact incidence and prevalence of CRPS after hand surgery is unknown, the reported incidence of CRPS is 5.5 to 26.2 per 100,000 person years, and the prevalence is reported as 20.7 per 100,000 person years.[1,2] Women are more frequently affected than men, with a ratio of 3:1 to 4:1; the upper extremity is involved more frequently than the lower extremity; and fracture is the most common causative event.[1,2] The following rates of upper extremity CRPS have been reported: 4.5% to 40% after fasciectomy for Dupuytren contracture,[3] 2% to 5% after carpal tunnel surgery,[4,5] and 22% to 39% after distal radius fracture.[6]

Current dogma states that early recognition and treatment of CRPS improves the prognosis for full recovery; however, the term "early" is not well defined. In a population-based study in Olmsted County, 74 patients were diagnosed with CRPS type I between 1989 and 1999 and 74% of these cases "resolved."[2] Another study that followed outcomes after distal radius fractures found that the stiffness noted at 12 weeks ("early" diagnosis of CRPS) correlated with residual symptoms at 10 years.[7] In addition, individuals who smoke have a poor prognosis compared with nonsmokers.[8]

DIAGNOSIS

CRPS is a clinical syndrome without a pathognomonic marker. CRPS type 1, also known as classic reflex sympathetic dystrophy, is defined as chronic pain without identifiable nerve involvement. CRPS type 2, also known as causalgia, includes pain with identified nerve involvement. In addition to pain, both syndromes are often associated with autonomic dysfunction (abnormal vasomotor activity, inappropriate piloerector activity, abnormal sweat gland activity, and inappropriate arteriovenous shunting) and functional impairment. Trophic changes may occur but vary with the severity of the precipitating event, the time after injury, or the degree of extremity compromise.

Department of Orthopaedic Surgery, Wake Forest University School of Medicine, Wake Forest University Health Sciences, Medical Center Boulevard, Winston-Salem, NC 27157, USA
* Corresponding author.
E-mail address: bpsmith@wfubmc.edu

Hand Clin 26 (2010) 281–289
doi:10.1016/j.hcl.2009.11.001

HISTORY AND PHYSICAL EXAMINATION

In patients diagnosed with postoperative CRPS, the details of the initiating injury or process are critical in developing a management plan. Therefore, the events leading to surgery should be reviewed to ascertain any preexisting conditions, past traumatic injuries or pain issues, and preexisting subclinical problems; all these variables may affect symptoms that occur after the surgery. For example, for patients with mild compression neuropathies (eg, carpal tunnel syndrome), quiescent CRPS may be exacerbated in the perioperative period and serve as a neuropathic event. Concomitant injuries or preexisting mechanical derangements may also potentiate nociceptive stimulation and contribute to the dystrophic process. There are no firm temporal relationships between the time of injury and the time of surgery, that is, early or late intervention has not been demonstrated to affect the incidence of CRPS.

The time of onset of CRPS after surgery varies, with symptoms appearing as early as in the post-anesthesia care unit (recovery room) or several weeks after surgery. Similar to nonsurgically related CRPS, the presentation may be obvious, with severe classic pain and swelling, or it may be insidious. Symptoms of CRPS are often nonspecific; pain, numbness, swelling, and stiffness are the normal symptoms reported by most postoperative patients. Therefore, clinical vigilance and acumen are crucial to discern CRPS within the context of nonspecific symptoms and signs and to evaluate the responses of these symptoms to the treatment and the passage of time. Recognizing the clinical character of CRPS is often crucial. In a classic presentation, this character includes pain that (1) is often described as burning, throbbing, and searing; (2) does not respond to narcotics; and (3) awakens patients at night or prevents normal sleep. Patients with CRPS are irritable and have difficulty with rehabilitation programs. In subtle or indolent presentations of CRPS, patients are often described as "uncooperative." They may complain of stiffness, swelling, cold sensitivity, hyperalgesia, and allodynia. Return to work or normal activities is resisted, and patients may appear listless and forlorn. They are often irritated by family, coworkers, and medical providers, and this feeling is often mutual. In contrast, patients who present with massive swelling of their extremity, especially associated with a zone of demarcation, multiple sores, unexplainable wound breakdown, and/or abnormal hand clenching, need to be evaluated carefully to rule out a diagnosis of a fictitious disorder or malingering.[9] However, CRPS is not a psychiatric disease and is not related to any known psychological profile.[6] Because CRPS is, in effect, an abnormal prolongation of normal physiologic responses to injury in the periphery, in the spinal cord, and throughout the central nervous system, there is the potential for it to occur in any patient after surgical intervention.

PHYSICAL EXAMINATION

The physical examination of patients suspected of having postsurgical CRPS should be compared with their preoperative examination. Tight wound dressings or casts should be avoided. The examination needs to assess from the neck to the fingers, including all aspects of the affected extremity. The extremity inspection should include palpation; assessments of skin integrity, range of motion, joint stability, and motor power; and neurologic, vascular, and sensibility assessments. The extremity examination should also assess stiffness, edema, atrophy of hair and nails, hypersensitivity, and dexterity. Hand and extremity postures should be observed at rest and during activity or gait. Neuropathic or nociceptive contributors to the pain process should be investigated and identified. New exacerbations of preexisting subclinical compression neuropathy should be evaluated by motor examination, sensory testing, and mechanical indications (ie, Tinel signs).

Part of the physical examination should be focused on the identification of possible nerve injuries. Carpal tunnel syndrome may occur after distal radial fracture surgery or hand/wrist reconstruction, and it may require nonoperative or operative treatment. Iatrogenic nerve injury with neuromas-in-continuity and neuromas or perineural irritation of mixed nerves or sensory branches can also act as powerful drivers of CRPS. Commonly reported nerve injuries associated with CRPS include those that are associated with the palmar cutaneous branch of the median nerve, the superficial radial nerve and its branches, and the dorsal branch of the ulnar nerve and its branches. However, injury or irritation of any nerve can contribute to a dystrophic process.

Inspection and Observation

The hands of patients with CRPS may be swollen, obscuring the dorsal veins, and/or the hands may appear dry or damp; the posture of the hand is generally intrinsic minus (metacarpophalangeal [MP] joints extended and proximal interphalangeal [PIP] joint slightly flexed). Dystonia, posturing, or tremors are also occasionally observed. For a thorough examination, the upper limb should be observed at rest, during activity, and during ambulation. Surgical sites should be inspected for signs of wound infection or surgical complications that vary from the expected usual complications.

Palpation

Patients may experience hyperpathia, allodynia, numbness, or hyperalgesia. Therefore, it is important to palpate the arm and hand to determine if these symptoms have a dermatomal distribution or if they are diffuse. If the symptoms are diffuse, the patient should be reevaluated after sympatholytic treatment.

Skin Integrity

The skin and any wounds around the affected area should be assessed carefully for signs of altered sensibility, abnormal autonomic function, and trophic changes.

Motor Testing

An evaluation of motor power must be performed to determine if there are weakness or endurance issues. Computerized endurance testing may be beneficial for collecting this information. Both intrinsic and extrinsic motor testing must be evaluated.

Range of Motion

The range of motion of all joints, including the shoulder, should be evaluated and recorded. Adhesive capsulitis or restricted range of motion of the shoulder is common in patients with long-standing CRPS. In patients with long-standing CRPS of the hand, intrinsic muscle contractures are also common. Therefore, the hand should be evaluated for any evidence of contracture.

Joint Stability

Joints should be assessed for global stability. Joint instability may elicit or contribute to nociceptive stimuli that contribute to CRPS. Instability of ulno-humeral, radiohumeral, distal radioulnar, radiocarpal, intercarpal, and finger joints may all contribute to significant nociception. In addition, tears in the triangular fibrocartilage complex or chronic sprains and strains may contribute to CRPS.

Neurologic Examination

A careful neurologic examination should be performed to identify any possible neuropathic involvement, especially spinal cord or brachial plexus involvement. In addition, the patient should be evaluated for movement disorders, such as dystonia.

Vascular Examination

Vascular examination is important to identify any vascular deficiencies and should not be neglected.

Sensibility Examination

Assessments of pain threshold (monofilaments) and innervation density (2-point discrimination) may be beneficial and can suggest a neuropathic component to the pain syndrome (CRPS type 2).

DIAGNOSTIC EVALUATION
Mechanical Testing

Pain threshold evaluations may be performed using algometers, dolorimeters, computer-assisted stimulation devices, and thermal threshold machines.[10] It is difficult to obtain these evaluations except in large medical centers; however, when available, they provide clinically useful, objective information. Von Frey monofilaments can also be used to determine pain thresholds.

Autonomic Function Evaluation

Autonomic function of the hands may be assessed by an evaluation of vasomotor control after the application of a stressor (ie, exposure to cold) as part of an isolated cold stress testing.[5] Sweat production may be determined by measuring resting sweat output and by the quantitative sudomotor axon reflex test.[11] Thermography, when used with a physiologic stressor, provides valuable confirmatory information.[12] These tests provide objective measures of autonomic function; however, they are only available at selected tertiary referral centers.

Radiologic Testing

Many investigators have recommended 3-phase bone scans as a diagnostic tool for CRPS. Positive scan results support the clinical diagnosis of CRPS. A positive 3-phase bone scan result in patients with CRPS is characterized by increased third phase bone scan periarticular uptake in all joints. Evidence of vasomotor instability and abnormal patterns of flow distribution may also be evident on phase I and phase II bone scans. However, these scans document vasomotor abnormalities, and therefore, they are not diagnostic for CRPS. The difficulty in using bone scans as a diagnostic tool for CRPS is that the scans may have insufficient sensitivity and specificity in patients with partially treated CRPS or in patients with variant presentations of the syndrome. These findings have led to Lee and Week's[13] analysis of the existing literature and their conclusion that "a three phase bone scan is not a prerequisite for the diagnosis of complex regional pain syndrome." Quantitative scintigraphies (bone scans) have demonstrated that there are both cortical and cancellous osteopenia that appear in excess of that observed with entry-matched controls treated with casting.[14]

Sympatholytic Challenge Testing

Sympathetically maintained pain (SMP) may be differentiated from sympathetically independent pain by a sympatholytic challenge provided by an intravenous injection of phentolamine, which is a combination of α_1- and α_2-adrenergic receptor blockers. In patients with SMP, the injection results in transient pain relief.[15] Similarly, stellate ganglion blocks, single cervical epidural blocks, sympathetic brachial plexus blocks, or scalene blocks may provide temporary relief of pain in patients with SMP. In patients who respond during the block, pain is relieved, whereas motor function remains. Although single blocks provide a useful diagnostic test, they are associated with significant false-negative rates. However, they are helpful in differentiating patients with SMP from patients with sympathetically independent pain.

TREATMENT

Early recognition of CRPS and the prompt initiation of treatment seems to improve patient outcomes. However, diagnosis and treatment of CRPS within 6 to 12 weeks of the onset of symptoms is not common in most patients; delays in diagnosis and treatment are especially common in patients with milder variants of CRPS. In addition, patients who develop CRPS after fractures, especially of the distal radius, seem to have a worse prognosis even when the CRPS is discovered early and treated promptly.

Treatment decisions are guided by the patients' symptoms and whether their pain is sympathetically maintained or sympathetically independent. In addition, the presence of an identifiable nociceptive or neuropathic component may require surgical intervention. Treatment is often multifactorial and involves a combination of therapy, oral medications, parenteral medications, and surgery. Hand therapy and various treatment modalities are usually combined with oral medications. Commonly, hand therapy including active and passive range of motion, splinting, and contrast baths (alternating heat and cold) is used. Other interventions that are beneficial for some patients are transcutaneous nerve stimulators, H-wave therapy, and stress loading.[10]

Oral pharmacologic intervention is used frequently to manage the symptoms of CRPS.

Currently, there are no drugs for CRPS that are labeled by the Federal Drug Administration (FDA), and few drugs are approved for chronic neuropathic pain. However, based on clinical experience and the literature, the following classes of drugs with a sympatholytic component have been recommended for use in patients with CRPS: antidepressants, anticonvulsants, membrane stabilizing agents, and adrenergic agents. The most common oral agents in these categories are listed in **Table 2**. The types of oral medications that are prescribed depend, in part, on the patient's presentation. For a hot, swollen hand, an antidepressant combined with an anticonvulsant is prescribed in conjunction with hand therapy. Commonly used drugs include a tricyclic antidepressant in low doses (ie, amitriptyline [Elavil], 25 mg three times a day, or amitriptyline, 50 mg, at bedtime for a normal-sized adult) combined with phenytoin (Dilantin), 100 mg three times a day, or pregabalin (Lyrica), 75 to 100 mg twice a day or three times a day. For patients with cold, stiff hands, a mild antidepressant is often combined with a calcium channel blocker. Another common drug regimen is amitriptyline combined with amlodipine (Norvasc).

For patients with acute hyperalgesia or allodynia and mild to moderate edema, an adrenergic agent (eg, clonidine [Catapres]) may be of benefit. A clonidine patch (0.1 mg) is applied over the most sensitive area; the application of the patches is combined with hand therapy, including a stress loading program. Steroid dose packs are used by many physicians and have demonstrated efficacy in reducing symptoms. Corticosteroids act to stabilize membranes and to decrease inflammatory pain (**Table 1**).

Prophylactic Treatment

Vitamin C taken prophylactically at a dose of 500 mg/d has been shown to decrease the incidence of CRPS in patients who sustain distal radius fractures.[16] However, the role of other vitamins in the treatment of CRPS is unclear.

Parenteral Agents

Generally, parenteral agents are administered by anesthesiologists. However, recent controlled studies have not demonstrated the efficacy of intravenous treatment of CRPS.[17,18] Intravenous agents, such as guanethidine, cortisone, reserpine, lidocaine, and bretylium, have been used previously. Of these drugs, bretylium tosylate was the only drug labeled by the FDA for this

Table 1
Definitions

Nociception	Detection of an unpleasant (noxious) stimulus that produces pain in human subjects under normal circumstances
Allodynia	Pain in a specific dermatomal or autonomous distribution associated with light touch to the skin; a stimulus that is not normally painful
Hyperalgesia	Increased sensitivity to pain (includes allodynia and hyperesthesia)
Hyperesthesia	Increased sensitivity to stimulation (pain on response to a mild nonnoxious stimulus)
Sympathetic pain	Pain in the presence of and/or associated with over action of the sympathetic pain fibers; by definition, the pain is relieved by sympatholytic interventions
Hypoesthesia	Decreased sensitivity to stimulation
Hyperpathia	Abnormally painful reaction to a stimulus (especially repetitive); often includes extended duration of pain, frequently with a delay
Dysesthesia	An unpleasant, abnormal sensation
Paresthesia	An abnormal sensation

purpose; however, marketing of bretylium in the United States has been discontinued.

Epidural clonidine and corticosteroids have been used successfully in patients with refractory symptoms.[19,20] The blockade may be achieved by indwelling catheters located in the epidural space or contiguous with portions of the brachial plexus or peripheral nerves. These continuous blocks may be used for 1 to 5 days as an outpatient treatment when used to target peripheral nerves.

Some of the newer treatments for CRPS include the use of free radical scavengers, including dimethyl sulfoxide, vitamin C, and N-acetyl-cysteine.[16,21] Their mechanism of action is hypothesized to be related to their ability to interfere with oxygen radical–mediated inflammatory response.[22] Calcitonin,[23] bisphosphonates,[24–26] and N-methyl-D-asparate antagonists (eg, ketamine, memantine)[27,28] have been used to treat patients with CRPS, with reported reduction in symptoms. However, controlled trials will be required to determine the efficacy of these drugs.

Surgical Treatment

Surgery to correct neuropathic or nociceptive sites plays an important role in the treatment of patients with CRPS. If indicated, surgery may be performed early if the CRPS symptoms cannot be controlled medically. The dictum that surgery is inappropriate and doomed to failure in patients with CRPS is incorrect and deprives patients of valuable and necessary interventions. However, surgical procedures should be used with caution, and care should be taken in determining the appropriate choice of surgical intervention. Before surgery, it is important to confirm that the pain is predominantly SMP and that it can be controlled with medications or continuous blocks.

Surgery to release compressed nerves, to correct or cushion neuromas-in-continuity, or to relieve perineural fibrosis may offer significant benefits to some patients.[29,30] Another option, the surgical ablation of sympathetic nerves by reversible means, such as phenol injections or radiofrequency ablation, may provide symptom relief. In other patients, neurolysis and blockade of peripheral nerves may be efficacious. Spinal cord stimulation provides effective pain relief in 50% of patients.[31] Use of implantable nerve stimulators and dorsal column stimulators are valuable as salvage procedures in selected patients with refractory symptoms.[6,32,33] Other salvage procedures for the most difficult cases include the use of dorsal column stimulators and gray matter stimulators and cingulotomy.[34]

Psychological Treatment

Counseling, biofeedback, and adaptive therapy can be beneficial for certain patients with CRPS. Although CRPS is not a psychiatric disease, chronic pain does affect health-related quality of life. Patients with CRPS may experience reactive depression as a result of their symptoms.

LATE MANAGEMENT OF COMPLICATIONS RELATED TO CRPS

Surgery on the extremities of patients with CRPS is appropriate if pain cannot be managed using other methods. Assuming that perioperative pain control is possible using sympatholytic interventions,

Table 2
Oral medications

Drug	Usual Dosage	Mechanism	Major Short-Term Disadvantage or Side Effects	Contraindications
Amitriptyline hydrochloride (Elavil)	25 mg tid or 50 mg qhs	Inhibits amine pump-decreased norepinephrine reuptake	Drowsiness	With guanethidine sulfate
Amlodipine (Norvasc)	5–10 mg qd	Ca^{++} channel blocking agent; prevents arteriovenous shunting; increases nutritional flow	Headache Postural hypotension	
Corticosteroids	20–80 mg/d; prednisone equivalents × 5–40 d	Stabilizes membranes; increases nutritional flow; decreases inflammatory pain	Adrenal suppression Avascular necrosis (dose related)	
Fluoxetine (Prozac)	20 mg/d AM	Serotonin reuptake inhibitor	Minimal drowsiness	
Gabapentin (Neurontin)	300–600 mg tid		Dizziness Somnolence Ataxia	Renal disease; patients must be carefully monitored
Nifedipine (Procardia)	10 mg tid, may increase slowly to 30 mg tid	Ca^{++} channel blocking agent; prevents arteriovenous shunting; increases nutritional flow	Headache Postural hypotension	
Phenoxybenzamine hydrochloride (Dibenzyline)	40–120 mg/d	α_1-receptor blocking agent	Orthostatic hypotension	
Phenytoin (Dilantin)	100 mg tid	Decreases resting membrane potentials; inhibits amine pump; stabilizes synaptic membrane	Ataxia Liver damage Convulsion	Liver disease Pregnancy
Pregabalin (Lyrica)	50–200 mg tid		Dizziness Somnolence Peripheral edema	

nociceptive and neuropathic foci may be managed by appropriate neurolysis of compressed nerves, repair of damaged nerves, or perineural fibrosis in correction of mechanical lesions. In addition, patients with CRPS may develop MP and PIP joint contractures that can be managed by surgical release. Contracted intrinsic muscles are common in these patients, and intrinsic releases may be beneficial. In addition, bony malunion or nonunion may occur because of the CRPS-induced osteopenia. For these patients, osteotomies may be warranted to gain the necessary correction. Neuropathic foci are managed using the same techniques that are used for patients with neuropathic foci without CRPS. Nerve repair, neurolysis, nerve wrapping, resection of neuromas, and temporary blockade with phenol or cryoablation are various techniques that can be used successfully in these patients.

SPECIFIC ENTITIES
Distal Radius Fracture

The reported incidence of CRPS after distal radius fracture ranges from 2% to 39% and is one of the leading causes of poor outcomes and malpractice claims.[6] The incidence of CRPS is increased as a result of improper casting. The presence of CRPS and the resultant osteoporosis (in excess of similarly treated non-CRPS fracture) contributes to delayed healing and nonunion. The delay in healing and the occurrence of nonunion is secondary to bone demineralization.[14] Onset of CRPS after distal radius fracture is variable and often delayed; stiffness, difficulty sleeping, burning pain, and cold sensitivity are the common symptoms. Median nerve involvement, often slow and insidious, may provide a neuropathic component, and for these patients, surgical release of the median nerve may be beneficial. In patients who are treated with external fixators or who have radial incisions, irritation or injury of the superficial radial nerve may create a neuropathic focus. Overdistraction, radioulnar joint instability, intercarpal instability, unstable triangular fibrocartilage complex, and/or chondral injury may contribute as nociceptive drivers of the pain process.

The most common presentation of CRPS after distal radius fracture is a warm, swollen hand; hyperpathia or allodynia; stiffness in which edema is responsive to elevation; and pain that is refractory to narcotics. The hot, swollen presentation usually occurs at 1 to 3 days after surgery, with associated median nerve symptoms reported by many patients. A more problematic alternative presentation of CRPS occurs when pain and stiffness are the predominate symptoms. The extremities of these patients are often cool, and swelling may be minimal. Patient compliance is compromised if active range of motion is restricted. These patients tend to request additional narcotics, and acquiescence to their demands by their treating physicians is rarely beneficial. Delayed union and osteopenia are often observed. Phase I and phase II bone scans may show hyperperfusion (hot/warm hand) and hypoperfusion (cool stiff hand); 3-phase scans show increased uptake at the fracture site and in the periarticular areas of the hand and wrist.

In patients with CRPS after distal radius fractures, awareness of the vagaries of presentation is crucial. Because the onset of CRPS may occur later, patients may develop symptoms during the 2- to 3-week period between their scheduled follow-up physician appointments. Therefore, office staff and other providers (especially nurses, nurse practitioners, physician assistants, and therapists) need to understand the importance of early diagnosis of CRPS based on symptoms reported by the patients. In patients reporting pain and stiffness, a chart notation that addresses the presence or absence of CRPS is an important safeguard. If CRPS is suspected, this concern should be noted, a sympatholytic medication should be prescribed, and consultation with a physician should be arranged. In patients who have coexistent carpal tunnel neuropathy, neurolysis of the median nerve should be performed.

Carpal Tunnel Surgery and CRPS

Severe chronic pain that occurs after carpal tunnel release surgery is classified as type 2 or neuropathic CRPS. In this instance, CRPS may be associated with nerve irritations related to the procedure (idiopathic), perineural fibrosis, or nerve injury (neuropraxia, neuromas-in-continuity, nerve transection). Onset of symptoms may be rapid, and patient symptoms can be apparent in the recovery room. However, in most cases, symptoms occur at 1 to 3 weeks after surgery. Injury to the palmar cutaneous nerve branch may occur and may be problematic in patients with coexistent CRPS. Patients present with pain, cold sensitivity, variable swelling, and difficulty sleeping. Nonsurgical management is the first line of treatment; however, for patients with refractory SMP, surgical intervention may be needed after an appropriate period of medical intervention fails to control pain.

If CRPS symptoms are only partially resolved after combinations of oral or parenteral pharmacologic treatment and therapy, surgery for neuropathic CRPS may be considered. Treatment options for perineural fibrosis include: (1) neurolysis alone,

(2) neurolysis and nerve wrapping, (3) neurolysis and local adipose transposition, and (4) neurolysis and muscle or fascial transposition or flaps. In the case of nerve injury, the injured nerves may be explored and neuromas may be repaired, resected, or transposed. However, palmar cutaneous nerve injuries are often difficult to repair. For the cases in which nerve repair is not possible, resection within soft tissue muscle implantation or grafting into an uninjured area is an option. As a salvage procedure, implantable nerve stimulations are available.[35]

Mechanical Derangements/Arthritis/ Cartilage Injury

Nociceptive events that contribute to dystrophic processes include intercarpal dissociations, osteochondral fractures with loose bodies, radiocarpal subluxation, triangular fibrocartilage complex injury, distal radioulnar joint instability, and chondrolysis. If symptoms are controlled incompletely by nonoperative interventions, surgery is appropriate to address these mechanical events.

SUMMARY

CRPS after hand surgery is not uncommon and may complicate postoperative care. Early diagnosis and treatment of CRPS is critical for optimal patient outcomes.

REFERENCES

1. de Mos M, de Bruijn AG, Huygen FJ, et al. The incidence of complex regional pain syndrome: a population-based study. Pain 2007;129(1–2):12–20.
2. Sandroni P, Benrud-Larson LM, McClelland RL, et al. Complex regional pain syndrome type I: incidence and prevalence in Olmsted County, a population-based study. Pain 2003;103(1–2):199–207.
3. Reuben SS. Preventing the development of complex regional pain syndrome after surgery. Anesthesiology 2004;101(5):1215–24.
4. Lichtman DM, Florio RL, Mack GR. Carpal tunnel release under local anesthesia: evaluation of the outpatient procedure. J Hand Surg Am 1979;4(6):544–6.
5. MacDonald RI, Lichtman DM, Hanlon JJ, et al. Complications of surgical release for carpal tunnel syndrome. J Hand Surg Am 1978;3(1):70–6.
6. Koman LA, Poehling GG, Smith BP, et al. Complex regional pain syndrome. In: Green D, Hotchkiss R, Pederson W, et al, editors. Green's operative hand surgery. 5th edition. Philadelphia: Churchill Livingstone; 2005. p. 2015–44.
7. Field J, Warwick D, Bannister GC. Features of algodystrophy ten years after Colles' fracture. J Hand Surg Br 1992;17:318–20.
8. An HS, Hawthorne KB, Jackson WT. Reflex sympathetic dystrophy and cigarette smoking. J Hand Surg Am 1988;13:470–2.
9. Grunert BK, Devine CA, Sanger JR, et al. Thermal self-regulation for pain control in reflex sympathetic dystrophy syndrome. J Hand Surg Am 1990;15:615–8.
10. Li Z, Smith BP, Smith TL, et al. Diagnosis and management of complex regional pain syndrome complicating upper extremity recovery. J Hand Ther 2005;18(2):270–6.
11. Chelimsky TC, Low PA, Naessens JM, et al. Value of autonomic testing in reflex sympathetic dystrophy. Mayo Clin Proc 1995;70(11):1029–40.
12. Bruehl S, Lubenow TR, Nath H, et al. Validation of thermography in the diagnosis of reflex sympathetic dystrophy. Clin J Pain 1996;12(4):316–25.
13. Lee GW, Weeks PM. The role of bone scintigraphy in diagnosing reflex sympathetic dystrophy. J Hand Surg Am 1995;20(3):458–63.
14. Bickerstaff DR, Kanis JA. Algodystrophy: an under-recognized complication of minor trauma. Br J Rheumatol 1994;33:240–8.
15. Raja SN, Treede RD, Davis KD, et al. Systemic alpha-adrenergic blockade with phentolamine: a diagnostic test for sympathetically maintained pain. Anesthesiology 1991;74(4):691–8.
16. Zollinger PE, Tuinebreijer WE, Breederveld RS, et al. Can vitamin C prevent complex regional pain syndrome in patients with wrist fractures? A randomized, controlled, multicenter dose-response study. J Bone Joint Surg Am 2007;89(7):1424–31.
17. Lake AP. Intravenous regional sympathetic block: past, present and future? Pain Res Manag 2004;9(1):35–7.
18. Livingstone JA, Atkins RM. Intravenous regional guanethidine blockade in the treatment of post-traumatic complex regional pain syndrome type 1 (algodystrophy) of the hand. J Bone Joint Surg Br 2002;84(3):380–6.
19. Dirksen R, Rutgers MJ, Coolen JM. Cervical epidural steroids in reflex sympathetic dystrophy. Anesthesiology 1987;66(1):71–3.
20. Rauck RL, Eisenach JC, Jackson K, et al. Epidural clonidine treatment for refractory reflex sympathetic dystrophy. Anesthesiology 1993;79(6):1163–9.
21. Perez RS, Zuurmond WW, Bezemer PD, et al. The treatment of complex regional pain syndrome type I with free radical scavengers: a randomized controlled study. Pain 2003;102(3):297–307.
22. Oyen WJ, Arntz IE, Claessens RM, et al. Reflex sympathetic dystrophy of the hand: an excessive inflammatory response? Pain 1993;55(2):151–7.
23. Hamamci N, Dursun E, Ural C, et al. Calcitonin treatment in reflex sympathetic dystrophy: a preliminary study. Br J Clin Pract 1996;50(7):373–5.
24. Manicourt DH, Brasseur JP, Boutsen Y, et al. Role of alendronate in therapy for posttraumatic complex

regional pain syndrome type I of the lower extremity. Arthritis Rheum 2004;50(11):3690–7.

25. Robinson JN, Sandom J, Chapman PT. Efficacy of pamidronate in complex regional pain syndrome type I. Pain Med 2004;5(3):276–80.

26. Varenna M, Zucchi F, Ghiringhelli D, et al. Intravenous clodronate in the treatment of reflex sympathetic dystrophy syndrome. A randomized, double blind, placebo controlled study. J Rheumatol 2000; 27(6):1477–83.

27. Goldberg ME, Domsky R, Scaringe D, et al. Multiday low dose ketamine infusion for the treatment of complex regional pain syndrome. Pain Physician 2005;8(2):175–9.

28. Sinis N, Birbaumer N, Gustin S, et al. Memantine treatment of complex regional pain syndrome: a preliminary report of six cases. Clin J Pain 2007; 23(3):237–43.

29. Jupiter JB, Seiler JG III, Zienowicz R. Sympathetic maintained pain (causalgia) associated with a demonstrable peripheral-nerve lesion. Operative

treatment. J Bone Joint Surg Am 1994;76(9):1376–84.

30. Koman LA, Smith BP, Smith TL. Stress testing in the evaluation of upper-extremity perfusion. Hand Clin 1993;9(1):59–83.

31. Taylor RS, Van Buyten JP, Buchser E. Spinal cord stimulation for complex regional pain syndrome: a systematic review of the clinical and cost-effectiveness literature and assessment of prognostic factors. Eur J Pain 2006;10(2):91–101.

32. Barolat G, Schwartzmann R, Woo R. Epidural spinal cord stimulation in the management of reflex sympathetic dystrophy. Appl Neurophysiol 1987;50:442–3.

33. Nashold BS Jr, Friedman H. Dorsal column stimulation for control of pain. J Neurosurg 1972;36:590–7.

34. Santo JL, Arias LM, Barolat G, et al. Bilateral cingulumotomy in the treatment of reflex sympathetic dystrophy. Pain 1990;41(1):55–9.

35. Strege DW, Cooney WP, Wood MB, et al. Chronic peripheral nerve pain treated with direct electrical nerve stimulation. J Hand Surg Am 1994;19(6):931–9.

Microsurgical Complications in the Upper Extremity

Jaimie T. Shores, MD*, W.P. Andrew Lee, MD

KEYWORDS

- Microsurgery • Replantation • Free tissue transfer
- Free flap • Complication • Thrombosis

Microsurgical complications are some of the most frustrating and potentially devastating complications that hand surgeons face. Complications may take the form of a complete or partial flap necrosis or loss of a revascularized or replanted part. One of the most frustrating scenarios is watching the slow dwindling demise of a replantation or free flap that is neither frankly necrotic nor functional. Despite these complications, microsurgeons push the edge of what is feasibly reconstructable or replantable.

Most microsurgical failures can be attributed to errors in the chronological spectrum of preoperative planning and patient preparation, intra-operative patient management and technical execution, and post-operative patient management. Many disease processes, patient conditions, and errors span more than one of these chronological categories.

PREOPERATIVE PLANNING

Preoperative planning must include not only the reconstructive options for the deficit or defect in question but also the patient's ability to tolerate a lengthy procedure with physiologic demands that may require complex intraoperative management. Consideration of physiologic age more than absolute age, cardiac and respiratory conditions, comorbid illness (such as diabetes mellitus, obesity, tobacco use, coronary artery disease, peripheral vascular disease, coagulopathic states, previous surgical history, and previous reactions to anesthesia), and family history of coagulopathy and vasculitis should all be evaluated. The timing of the surgery should be considered within this context. For example, a 72-year-old man with a history of hypertension, unstable angina, and tobacco use who loses 2 fingers because of zone II amputation with a table saw may not be a candidate for an emergency replantation if the risk of a long emergency operation to his health is judged to be significant. However, the same patient who is 2 weeks status post avulsion injury to the dorsal hand and forearm and has had time for a cardiac workup, including catheterization or stress testing, control of blood pressure, and perioperative risk reduction by recent institution of β-blocking agents, may be an acceptable candidate for free flap coverage of exposed bone or tendons.

Preoperative planning must also include the appropriate anatomic evaluation of recipient and donor sites. Many injuries that result in the need for microsurgical replantation may also have large zones of injury to vascular recipient targets and may require preoperative angiography of the arterial and venous systems. Angiography can also be helpful in identifying patients who can be downstaged to local/regional flaps based on permissive anatomy, such as reversed forearm flaps for dorsal hand coverage. Evaluation of appropriate donor sites is also crucial. Care should be taken in evaluating the functional and aesthetic needs of the reconstruction with the available donor sites to determine if the patient needs a muscle flap, myocutaneous flap, fascial flap with skin grafting,

Division of Plastic and Reconstructive Surgery, University of Pittsburgh School of Medicine, Suite 667, Scaife Hall, 3550 Terrace Street, Pittsburgh, PA 15261, USA
* Corresponding author.
E-mail address: shoresjt@upmc.edu

Hand Clin 26 (2010) 291–301
doi:10.1016/j.hcl.2010.01.007
0749-0712/10/$ – see front matter © 2010 Elsevier Inc. All rights reserved.

fasciocutaneous flap, or possibly even vascularized bone with coverage. Donor site considerations may include cosmetic appearance of the flap and the scar, hair growth, skin color match, and functional losses at the donor site (donor site morbidity).

Donor site considerations also include the size of the resultant defect and whether primary closure or skin grafting will be necessary. Pedicle length and vessel diameter must also be evaluated as one considers the location of microvascular anastamoses. Timing of operative intervention is also a relevant concern. Although revascularization/replantation may require an immediate operation to salvage the injured part, issues of coverage are usually more urgent than emergent. Godina[1] showed significantly improved flap survival when lower extremity defects were reconstructed within 72 hours. Francel and colleagues[2] then demonstrated that with a wide debridement and anastomoses performed on vessels not involved in the zone of injury, reconstruction could be expanded out to 15 days. Ofer and colleagues[3] had a different experience in extremity reconstruction for electrical injury. Flap survival was lowest in the 5 to 21 days range, and was 100% in the group delayed after 21 days. Further case series have since demonstrated safety with even more extended times of flap placement as long as debridements are thorough and vessels used for anastomoses are not considered within the zone of injury.[4] Most recently, Kumar and colleagues[5] evaluated their success with pedicled and free flap reconstruction of upper extremity wounds in war veterans from military operations in Iraq and Afghanistan. Despite times to closure that varied from weeks to months secondary to infection or other concomitant injuries, their flap survival rate (all flaps) was 96% with a 100% limb salvage rate.[5]

INTRAOPERATIVE CONSIDERATIONS

Anesthetic considerations and the surgeon's desires and expectations for the anesthesia team must be communicated effectively. All efforts to avoid hypotension and peripheral vasoconstriction or spasm must be taken. Patients must be well hydrated and resuscitated, warm, and comfortable. The use of vasopressors or inotropes should be avoided if possible. The authors require the anesthesia providers to clearly inform them in advance of any use of vasopressor or inotrope so that we have the option to abandon the reconstruction if the patient's condition will not tolerate blood pressure support by crystalloid and colloid alone.

Surgical execution must be goal oriented and disciplined. Inadequate debridement of the wound in question may result in postoperative infection, healing problems, or the inability to fully recognize the true nature of the wound and reconstructive needs. It may also prevent adequate recipient vessel preparation as a result of a lack of recognition of the zone of injury. Recipient vessel preparation is a critical step. Analysis of the fitness of the artery and vein or vena comitans (VCs) as recipient vessels should be made by the primary surgeon. Enough exposure to safely engage the recipient vessels is required. Overdissection should be avoided because this adds risk of vessel injury. Flap dissection should be meticulous but efficient. Prolonging the surgery because of extremely slow flap dissection only increases risks of hypothermia, fluid losses, vascular stasis, and intraoperative error caused by shift changes of staff and surgeon fatigue. Care must be taken to ensure that technically correct microsurgical anastomoses are performed without pedicle kinking, twisting or torsion, or compression on the pedicle. Pressure from vessel exposure site closure and flap inset should be guarded against. Vessel size discrepancies may be managed by changing the pedicle distance (longer pedicles may have larger vessels and vice versa), by microsurgical modification of the vessels themselves, or by performing end-to-side anastomoses.

Vascular grafting should be used whenever deemed necessary. Several groups have found that vein grafts are associated with higher free flap failure rates and bleeding.[6–10] However, especially in the case of replantation and revascularization, vein grafts may be absolutely critical in allowing microanastomoses to uninjured vessels, which otherwise would not support reperfusion. In a recent series of 103 lower-extremity free flap reconstructions, vein grafts were found to be indispensable and not related to flap loss, if performed with perfect technique.[11]

POSTOPERATIVE MANAGEMENT

The same factors considered in the intraoperative physiologic management of the patient must continue postoperatively. Patients must be kept warm, well hydrated, with their pain and anxiety controlled. Pain and sympathetic tone can frequently be dealt with by the placement of a peripheral anesthetic block catheter preoperatively, with continued postoperative use. The catheter must be checked frequently to ensure that it is still functioning adequately to prevent pain (unwanted hypertension, increased sympathetic tone, increased vasospasm) and unwanted patient movement. Dressings and positioning must be constantly checked to make sure that pressure, dependency, and tourniquet effect from bandages do not cause problems.

There is no universally-agreed-on flap monitoring system or schedule that has been demonstrated to be superior to all others. The authors use a combination of clinical evaluation and intermittent use of an implantable venous Doppler probe. There is no substitute for clinical evaluation by the surgeon for color, warmth, capillary refill, bleeding, and arterial and venous signal presence and quality. Patients with darker pigmentation may demonstrate a challenge to clinical monitoring of color and capillary refill. Patients with replants or revascularizations may benefit from placement of a pulse oximetry probe on the involved digit so that oxygen saturation and waveform may be compared with an uninjured digit.[12]

Care must be taken to avoid fluid overload in those without cardiopulmonary reserve where excess fluid could exacerbate conditions such as COPD or congestive heart failure. Young patients who are difficult to control in terms of postoperative thrashing and pain may benefit from a prolonged period of intubation and sedation in the intensive care unit (ICU) for the first 24 to 72 hours after surgery, during the most likely time period for flap complication.

EARLY COMPLICATIONS

Complications may present themselves as early as intraoperatively, with the inability to reperfuse the flap or a sudden loss of perfusion after a successful return of bleeding. Factors to consider include the overall ischemia time of the flap and the flap type. Muscle flaps with warm ischemia times of 3 hours or longer may suffer irreversible damage. Fascial and fasciocutaneous flaps are more tolerant to warm ischemia, providing twice the amount of time to irreversible injury. The irreversibly injured flap may demonstrate the "no-reflow" phenomenon whereby arterial inflow has been re-established but no venous outflow is demonstrated due to microcirculatory collapse.[13] This occurs through multiple mechanisms and is somewhat dependent upon actually re-establishing perfusion. As ischemia time progresses, endothelial cell injury and swelling occur. Reperfusion brings with it new oxygen free radicals which also contribute to further endothelial injury and activation prothrombotic cascades which ultimately result in narrowing of capillaries and small vessels, slowing of blood flow, further endothelial injury, inflammatory cell activation and margination, and microthrombi formation. Ultimately, after arterial in-flow is re-established, venous outflow is blocked at the microcirculation level, which eventually compromises flap in-flow as well.[14]

In the event that flap perfusion is unable to be restarted, the surgeon must reevaluate the vessel anastomoses, the pedicle position for kinking, torsion, or pressure, and the recipient artery and vein(s) for kinking, pressure, and to make sure that they have adequate inflow and outflow capability. Anastomoses may require revision, and if the recipient vessels appear damaged, another site may be required on the same vascular system or new recipient vessels. The pedicle vessels should be cleanly trimmed with each attempted anastomosis. Errors in planning may result in start of flap ischemia before recipient vessel preparation or recipient vessels that result in unfavorable pedicle geometry. If inflow and outflow problems are not the cause of poor flap perfusion, consider vessel spasm and check to make sure that the patient is normotensive and off vasopressors. Irrigate the vessels with vasodilators and the flap and vessels with warm saline.

Loss of perfusion in the early postoperative period is the most common reason for flap loss. Most vascular flap complications occur within the first 24 hours.[6,15,16] Loss of perfusion may be secondary to arterial or venous thrombosis. Pedicle compression may occur secondary to insetting of the flap too tight to accommodate for postoperative swelling. Compression may also be caused by hematoma, which can occur more commonly with vein grafts. The recognition of a compromised flap must be immediate if salvage efforts are to be successful. All bandages should be removed and sutures may be released at the bedside. The patient should be returned to the operating room as soon as possible. Salvage rates in the early period are directly related to how soon the compromised flap is recognized.[17,18]

LATE COMPLICATIONS

Flap loss after the first 72 hours is uncommon.[16,17] Furthermore, flap complications beginning 1 to 2 weeks postoperatively are even more unusual.[16] Most late complications are not related to the flap itself but to the host. Free flap operations may be long cases that increase risk of deep venous thrombosis (DVT) and subsequent pulmonary embolism. Risk factors for DVT include length of surgery, lower extremity trauma, and pelvic surgery. All patients who are able to be placed on mechanical prophylaxis (sequential compression devices, TED hose) and chemoprophylaxis (unfractionated heparin, low-molecular-weight heparin) should be meticulously and frequently checked to make sure that these measures are continuously being maintained in accordance with the American College of Chest Physicians' guidelines.[19,20]

Other complications may include pneumonia, fluid overload, acute renal failure, and infection related to exposed bone, joint, or hardware.

SPECIFIC FACTORS
Vessel Thrombosis

Vessel thrombosis is the most commonly thought of complication in microsurgery, occurring in 3.2% to 15% of all free tissue transfers.[6,15] Larger series, such as those by Bui and colleagues[17] and Nakatsuka and colleagues,[21] have pushed what had traditionally been rates of 10% to 15% down to 3.2% to 4%. Khouri and colleagues'[6] original series of 493 flaps demonstrated a 10% postoperative thrombosis rate, with an ultimate salvage of 69% of these threatened flaps resulting in an overall flap survival rate of 96%. In Nakatsuka and colleagues'[21] series of 2373 head and neck free flaps, arterial and venous thrombosis rates were roughly equal, totaling to 4% of all flaps performed. However, complete salvage rates were different for arterial and venous thromboses, 15% and 60% respectively. Bui and colleagues[17] demonstrated a salvage rate of 40% for arterial thrombosis and 71% for venous thromboses, with partial necrosis in 45% of the salvaged venous thromboses. Not frequently included in postoperative thrombosis rates are those thromboses that occur on the table during the initial flap transfer operation. These thromboses were originally reported by Khouri and colleagues[6] to be as high as 8% (41 flaps in a multicenter trial), with only 4.9% of that number (2 total flaps) going on to failure.

The timing of vessel thrombosis may differ from arteries to veins, but this has not been consistent. Khouri and colleagues showed that most arterial thromboses occurred within the first 24 hours, whereas venous thromboses predominated after 24 hours; however, Chen and colleagues[16] did not demonstrate the same findings. These investigators showed that arterial thromboses predominated after 48 hours and vascular complications after more than 1 week post operation were exclusively arterial in origin. All investigators demonstrated that most thromboses occur within the first 48 to 72 hours (Kroll and colleagues: 80% within 48 hours; Chen and colleagues: 95% within 72 hours). Chen and colleagues demonstrated that while arterial thromboses comprised 45.5% of flap occlusions their salvage rate was significantly less, being 75% versus 90% for venous problems.

Chen and colleagues also showed that in all compromised flaps, 51.3% demonstrated problems within the first 4 postoperative hours, whereas 82.3% of compromised flaps had been detected by 24 hours post operation, and 95.6% detected by 48 hours post operation.

Flap salvage rates are higher when the patient is taken back to the operating room sooner rather than later after detection (**Fig. 1**). Bui and colleagues[17] found improved flap survival when reexploration was accomplished within 4 hours of thrombosis detection versus after 9 hours; whereas Panchapakesan and colleagues[18] improved salvage when flaps were taken back within 1.9 hours versus after 4.1 hours. Flap perfusion may become clinically impaired even before a full vessel thrombosis has occurred, which further emphasizes the need for early take-back. Hidalgo and Jones[22] demonstrated no thromboses in flaps returned within 1.5 hours of detection and a 64% thrombosis rate if taken back after 3 hours.

Thrombosis salvage techniques may use traditional surgical techniques of anastomosis excision and revision, catheter thrombectomy, and pharmacologic thrombolysis. Streptokinase, urokinase, and recombinant tissue plasminogen activator (rTPA) have all been used for flap salvage after surgical/mechanical efforts to reestablish arterial or venous perfusion have failed. Neither streptokinase nor urokinase has a demonstrated advantage over the other in terms of efficacy in most studies,[23] but streptokinase has a demonstrated 6% risk of allergic reaction with 0.1% incidence of anaphylaxis.[24] Rinker and colleagues[25] have reported a retrospective review of flaps

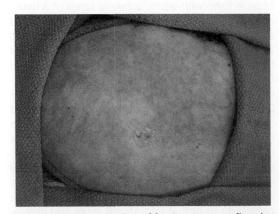

Fig. 1. Venous congestion of fasciocutaneous flap due to venous thrombosis. Thrombosis was detected quickly in this light skin colored flap, and the flap was successfully salvaged with immediate release of the VC to allow venous decompression and then reanastomosis.

salvaged with rTPA; a single 2.5-mg bolus and a second 2.5-mg bolus, only if no effect was observed. Ten of 15 flaps (67%) were salvaged in this manner.[25] These flaps were retrospectively compared with flap salvages attempted without rTPA, which had a success rate of only 29%. Systemic heparinization did not appear to affect outcome in this small study. Even catheter-directed rTPA thrombolysis has been described in a single arterial and a single venous thrombosis, with successful flap salvage.[26]

Replantations/Ring Avulsions

The decision to replant or revascularize an amputated part must be made quickly and with input from a well-educated patient or his or her family members, if possible. Salvage rates range from 66.3% to 90%, or better, depending on the mechanism and location of amputation.[27] In their series of 1018 replanted digits, Waikakul and colleagues[28] reported a 92% survival rate. Avulsion injuries have the lowest rate of success when salvage is attempted, with crush injuries performing only slightly better. The dogma that

Urbaniak grade III ring avulsions should not be replanted has recently been challenged (**Fig. 2**). Brooks and colleagues[29] demonstrated that type III avulsions can be replanted with an approximately 67% success rate and an ultimate total active motion of 174° and grip strength measuring 63% of the contralateral hand. The fate of microvascular anastomoses, even in successful replantations and revascularizations, is not straightforward. Once again, depending on mechanism, the digits' initial and long term survival rates do not necessarily reflect continued patency of repaired vessels. Lee and colleagues[30] demonstrated in 75 successfully replanted digits that by 15 days post operation, 37% of living digits had vessel occlusion. Occlusion varied by mechanism (clean guillotine type had the lowest rate: 8%) and by level of amputation. Despite this high occlusion rate, the digits continued to survive off new collateral flow through the healing skin margins.

More proximal amputations have more and higher risk-associated complications. When ultimate salvage of attempted replantations seems to be high, complications such as tissue necrosis and deep infection may be as well. Cavadas[31]

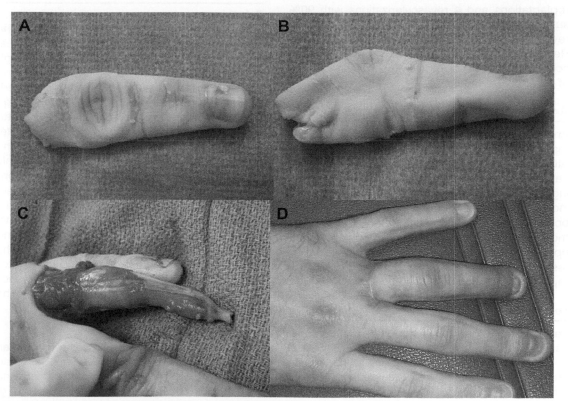

Fig. 2. Grade III ring avulsion injury. (*A*) and (*B*) Skin only envelop avulsion/amputation with nail plate and distal phalangeal tuft. (*C*) Ring finger with intact extensor and flexor mechanisms, note the distal phalangeal tuft fracture. (*D*) Viable digit undergoing therapy for range of motion (3 months post-operation).

described 56 amputations proximal to the wrist with 100% survival, but 11 demonstrated critical soft tissue necrosis or deep infection, requiring operative revision and pedicled or free flap coverage. More proximal replantations with skeletal muscle are less tolerant of ischemia and may require anatomic or extra-anatomic shunting of blood flow to salvage them during the initial surgery. Infection and necrosis may result from continuing demarcation and under-recognition of the need for more extensive debridement at the time of replantation.[32] The metabolic consequences of replantation must be considered so that further cardiovascular risk secondary to metabolic factors and renal failure secondary to direct and indirect factors do not put the patient at further risk. Close monitoring in an ICU setting for these complications is critical, as one published report discusses a life-saving re-amputation of a replanted arm due to systemic effects of ischemia-reperfusion injury.[32,33] In one series of 36 above elbow replantations, 4 patient deaths were noted secondary to multisystem organ failure due to the same processes and metabolic complications.[34]

Revision is the rule rather than the exception with replantation. Molski[35] reported a series of 18 replantations and 4 revascularizations with 90% survival. Of those who survived, 95% required revision, which significantly improved function. Revision procedures included nerve grafting, scar revision, tendon transfer, tenolysis, and repair of 1 vein graft aneurysm.

Aneurysm

Aneurysm, or more commonly, pseudoaneurysm, may complicate microsurgical anastomoses. Although this is a rare complication, aneurysm can rupture and cause substantial bleeding, risking the life of the flap and the patient. The exact incidence of aneurysms is unknown and it may occur within the first postoperative week, but more commonly between the ninth and 18th postoperative days.[36] It can be effectively treated by resection of the aneurysm and grafting or primary repair.

Leeching

Leeches have long been recognized as useful in salvaging pedicled flaps, free flaps, and replantations with venous insufficiency due to inadequate outflow. Indeed, several studies have cited their effectiveness in animal models and humans.[37–40] *Hirudo medicinalis* was approved as a medical device in the United States in 2004.[41] Complications from leeches consist of minor problems, such as leeches migrating to unwanted areas, especially when used around openings to anatomic cavities such as the nasopharynx, open sinuses, or cranial defects for which flaps are required. These defects may be protected with multiple types of "leech cages" or even with the judicious use of a suture being placed through the "tail" of the leech, which appears to not harm it or impede its ability to feed.[42,43] Other considerations are the need for frequent hemoglobin/hematocrit measurements, because patients will frequently require blood transfusion to compensate for continued bleeding from the area being leeched.[44] The most feared complication of leech use is infection. Incidences ranging from 2.4% to 20% have been reported, with clinical presentations ranging from cellulites, to abscess, to extensive soft tissue infections causing tissue loss and systemic sepsis.[45,46] Routine antimicrobial prophylaxis for *Aeromonas* species (usually *Aeromonas hyprophila*) and *Serratia marcescens* should be used. The most common agent recommended is a fluoroquinolone, although routine antibiotic practices vary.[47,48]

Specific Patient Factors

Tobacco use

Tobacco use is commonly encountered in the patient needing replantation and/or microsurgical reconstruction of the upper extremity. Although not a contraindication to emergency surgery, diminished outcomes from tobacco use are noted. Waikakul and colleagues[28] noted in their large series of digital replantations that cigarette smoking was associated with higher failure rate. Although their overall survival rate was 92%, the survival rate in smokers was found to be only 61%. However, several investigators have demonstrated equivalent survival of free flaps in smokers and nonsmokers. Although most of these results have been obtained in elective or semielective free flap surgeries, such as those for head and neck reconstruction or breast reconstruction, the effects of tobacco on their microvascular anastomoses seem to be nil.[6,49–51] However, wound-healing complications were demonstrated to be higher in smokers.[50,51]

Medical comorbidity

Age, obesity, and diabetes mellitus have not been demonstrated to have a direct effect on flap survival.[6,52,53] However, medical comorbidity and age require special consideration in terms of risk assessment and medical management, perioperatively and postoperatively, because donor-site complications may be higher in all of these patients. Medical morbidity has been shown to be significantly higher in octogenarians despite excellent flap survival and low surgical morbidity.[52]

Flap Type

Initial animal studies demonstrated a higher efficacy of muscle flaps in obliterating dead space and bringing new blood supply to contaminated wounds with hopes of preventing osteomyelitis or treating established osteomyelitis.[54,55] Clinical outcomes of lower extremity wounds treated with muscle flaps seemed to confirm the reported animal model efficacy.[55,56] However, fasciocutaneous flaps have been demonstrated to be equally efficacious in distal third lower extremity wounds.[57] These findings have been supported in laboratory animal models[58] and in patients with acute and chronic osteomyelitis.[59,60] The theoretical benefit of muscle flaps adding blood supply to a wound bed have only been demonstrated in flaps with a salvageable vascular complication, which stimulated angiogenesis within the wound bed. Machens and colleagues[61] demonstrated the dependence of flaps upon their pedicles and not on collateral circulation for as long as 10 years after the initial free flap procedure. However, muscle and fasciocutaneous flaps both seem to reintegrate lymphatic flow.[62]

Muscle flaps with skin grafts may be harder to salvage if a vascular complication occurs.[6] This may simply be because of the absence of a skin paddle for monitoring, which would enable earlier detection of failure.

SUMMARY

Most of the microvascular experience concerning free flap reconstruction of the upper extremity is based on microsurgical reconstruction of the head and neck, breast, and lower extremity, and much data applied to the upper extremity is therefore extrapolated. However, today the flap survival rates are high as long as preoperative, intraoperative, and postoperative factors are considered and optimized. No specific pharmacologic protocol has demonstrated superiority in flap survival. Factors to consider in ensuring flap survival should include the patient's overall condition, donor sites (in terms of flap source and morbidity), wound characteristics, reconstructive goals, need for further surgeries, and surgeon experience. Khouri and colleagues[6] stated in their 1998 prospective study on outcomes of microsurgery that, in addition to having experienced microsurgeons practicing at the high end of the microsurgery learning curve, "…The findings suggest that diligent intraoperative technique and observation, not postoperative pharmacologic treatment, can reduce the need for surgical take-back and resultant high flap failure rate." In essence, fastidious technique, experience, obsessive planning, and patient management are vital components to successful microsurgery, be it replantation or free flap reconstruction.

Illustrative Case

A 21-year-old right-handed African American male receives his second gunshot wound to the left forearm in 6 months, resulting in a segmental and comminuted fracture of the ulna with a 10 × 23 cm soft tissue defect with exposed hardware and ulna after debridement and open reduction internal fixation (**Fig. 3**). The patient is a heavy marijuana smoker but has no other significant medical history. Preoperative computed tomography (CT) angiography shows patency of his

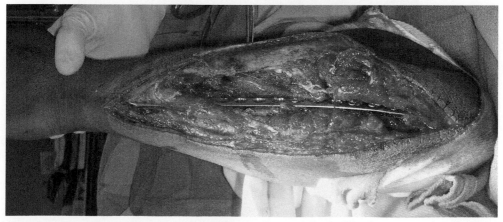

Fig. 3. Open gunshot wound to left forearm with exposed fixated ulna and hardware prior to debridement and coverage.

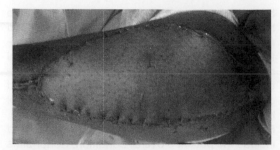

Fig. 4. ALT free flap on initial detection of venous thrombosis. Note the lack of striking color change as shown in **Fig. 1**.

radial and ulnar arteries and normal venous filling of his cephalic and basilic veins extending from the arm to the wrist. The patient undergoes free flap reconstruction with an ipsilateral anterolateral thigh (ALT) flap. Preoperative unfractionated heparin is given for DVT prophylaxis and repeated every 8 hours throughout the operation. An implantable venous Doppler is placed on the basilic vein proximal to the anastomosis of both VCs within the ALT pedicle. The patient is maintained on aspirin and DVT prophylaxis with low-molecular-weight heparin postoperatively. He is extubated and taken to the ICU for monitoring with an indwelling supraclavicular catheter for pain control and sympathetic blockade.

The flap has normal color and arterial signals within the cutaneous paddle until approximately 44 hours post operation when a venous signal is no longer detected via the implanted Doppler probe (**Fig. 4**). There are no color changes within the skin paddle and the flap still has arterial signals, albeit dampened and of a water-hammer quality. The patient reports that he began having more pain in his arm several hours before and has been moving his arm frequently in attempts to get comfortable. Bandages and sutures are removed at the bedside without change, and the patient is taken back to the operating room for emergent exploration.

In the operation room (OR), exploration of the pedicle reveals thrombosis of the basilic vein proximal to the site of anastomosis with soft clot extending into the VCs and into the perforators within the flap. Division of the VCs shows slow but incomplete expulsion of the soft clot. The clot is manually removed, with no restoration of venous outflow despite blunted arterial Doppler signals that are still present within the artery. The VCs are flushed with heparin, and 50 mg of rTPA is slowly infused into the ulnar artery just proximal to the arterial anastomosis and retrograde through the VCs over the course of 2 to 3 hours. Still no reflow is observed. A dermatome is used to harvest a split-thickness

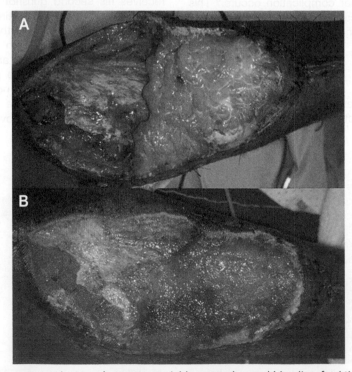

Fig. 5. Serial debridements continue to demonstrate viable appearing and bleeding fat (*A*). However, days later the same tissue appears desiccated and nonviable (*B*).

skin graft from the flap for tissue banking, which reveals multiple areas of dark venous bleeding from the dermis. At this point, the VCs are left uncoupled and a drain placed beneath the flap. Arterial signals and slow venous bleeding from the dermis are present, and the patient is sent to the ICU with institution of leech therapy with antibiotic prophylaxis. Hematology is consulted for hypercoagulability workup, which detects inherited protein S deficiency. Continued DVT prophylaxis is recommended with no contraindication for further microsurgery, if necessary.

After 36 hours, leeches stop attaching and no further bleeding is observed. The exposed dermis begins to dry and becomes eschar in patchy areas with preservation of more normal dermis in other areas. The flap is returned to the OR for debridement, which reveals viable appearing fat with bright red blood-filled capillaries that bleed when cut. A wound vacuum-assisted closure (VAC) is applied. Each time the wound VAC is changed, the superficial fat appears somewhat desiccated, whereas deeper fat appears healthy and viable with each debridement (**Fig. 5**). This process continues for approximately 10 days after the initial take-back. At this time, the banked skin graft is applied to the healthy-appearing fat and exposed portions of ALT fascia after multiple debridements.

After another week, the skin graft is adherent and viable over the grafted fascia but appears desiccated over the now darker fat of the flap directly over the exposed plate and bone. At this point, the entire flap and wound are debrided because it is clear that the patient's reconstruction is not salvageable. An immediate contralateral ALT flap is performed with anastomoses to the ulnar artery and ulnar VCs in a different area, with identical DVT prophylaxis measures intraoperatively. The patient is kept intubated and sedated for the 72 hours after the free flap operation to prevent agitation and limit damaging movement of the extremity that was observed after the first operation. The patient is maintained continuously on aspirin and low-molecular-weight heparin as he had been throughout his hospitalization.

Hyperpyrexia, mild hypertension, and tachycardia are observed throughout his ICU stay while intubated, believed to be secondary to his multiple medications that are required for sedation. On extubation, his fever abates and mild hypertension resolves, and he is transferred out of the ICU, but his tachycardia persists. The flap is viable with normal arterial and venous signals detected within the skin paddle. He has no signs of upper or lower extremity DVT on physical examination. A CT angiogram of the chest is ordered, which reveals bilateral non-flow limiting pulmonary emboli. Duplex studies fail to detect DVT within the neck, upper limbs, or lower extremities. A CT venogram is performed, which fails to identify an embolic source. The hematologist reevaluates, judging that the patient also possesses lupus anticoagulant, and recommends chronic coumadinization. On discharge, the patient has a viable flap (**Fig. 6**) with completed bony and soft tissue reconstruction, new diagnoses of protein S deficiency and Lupus anticoagulant, 6 months of coumadin therapy, but no clinically apparant sequalae of pulmonary embolus.

REFERENCES

1. Godina M. Early microsurgical reconstruction of complex trauma of the extremities. Plast Reconstr Surg 1986;78(3):285–92.
2. Francel TJ, Vander Kolk CA, Hoopes JE, et al. Microvascular soft-tissue transplantation for reconstruction of acute open tibial fractures: timing of coverage and long-term functional results. Plast Reconstr Surg 1992;89(3):478–87 [discussion: 479–88].
3. Ofer N, Baumeister S, Megerle K, et al. Current concepts of microvascular reconstruction for limb salvage in electrical burn injuries. J Plast Reconstr Aesthet Surg 2007;60(7):724–30.
4. Karanas YL, Nigriny J, Chang J. The timing of microsurgical reconstruction in lower extremity trauma. Microsurgery 2008;28(8):632–4.
5. Kumar AR, Grewal NS, Chung TL, et al. Lessons from the modern battlefield: successful upper extremity injury reconstruction in the subacute period. J Trauma 2009;67(4):752–7.
6. Khouri RK, Cooley BC, Kunselman AR, et al. A prospective study of microvascular free-flap surgery and outcome. Plast Reconstr Surg 1998;102(3): 711–21.
7. Miller MJ, Schusterman MA, Reece GP, et al. Interposition vein grafting in head and neck reconstructive microsurgery. J Reconstr Microsurg 1993;9(3): 245–51 [discussion: 251–2].
8. Buncke HJ, Alpert B, Shah KG. Microvascular grafting. Clin Plast Surg 1978;5(2):185–94.

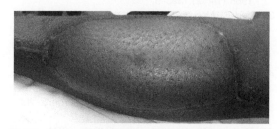

Fig. 6. Final reconstruction after complete debridement of previous flap and new ALT free flap placement.

9. Germann G, Steinau HU. The clinical reliability of vein grafts in free-flap transfer. J Reconstr Microsurg 1996;12(1):11–7.

10. Chaivanichsiri P. Influence of recipient vessels on free tissue transplantation of the extremities. Plast Reconstr Surg 1999;104(4):970–5.

11. Bayramicli M, Tetik C, Sonmez A, et al. Reliability of primary vein grafts in lower extremity free tissue transfers. Ann Plast Surg 2002;48(1):21–9.

12. Chang J, Jones N. Twelve simple maneuvers to optimize digital replantation and revascularization. Tech Hand Up Extrem Surg 2004;8(3):161–6.

13. Ames A 3rd, Wright RL, Kowada M, et al. Cerebral ischemia. II. The no-reflow phenomenon. Am J Pathol 1968;52(2):437–53.

14. Calhoun KH, Tan L, Seikaly H. An integrated theory of the no-reflow phenomenon and the beneficial effect of vascular washout on no-reflow. Laryngoscope 1999;109(4):528–35.

15. Kroll SS, Schusterman MA, Reece GP, et al. Timing of pedicle thrombosis and flap loss after free-tissue transfer. Plast Reconstr Surg 1996; 98(7):1230–3.

16. Chen KT, Mardini S, Chuang DC, et al. Timing of presentation of the first signs of vascular compromise dictates the salvage outcome of free flap transfers. Plast Reconstr Surg 2007;120(1):187–95.

17. Bui DT, Cordeiro PG, Hu QY, et al. Free flap reexploration: indications, treatment, and outcomes in 1193 free flaps. Plast Reconstr Surg 2007;119(7):2092–100.

18. Panchapakesan V, Addison P, Beausang E, et al. Role of thrombolysis in free-flap salvage. J Reconstr Microsurg 2003;19(8):523–30.

19. Nutescu EA. Assessing, preventing, and treating venous thromboembolism: evidence-based approaches. Am J Health Syst Pharm 2007;64(11 Suppl 7): S5–13.

20. Geerts WH, Bergqvist D, Pineo GF, et al. Prevention of venous thromboembolism: American College of Chest Physicians Evidence-Based Clinical Practice Guidelines (8th edition). Chest 2008;133(6 Suppl): 381S–453S.

21. Nakatsuka T, Harii K, Asato H, et al. Analytic review of 2372 free flap transfers for head and neck reconstruction following cancer resection. J Reconstr Microsurg 2003;19(6):363–8 [discussion: 369].

22. Hidalgo DA, Jones CS. The role of emergent exploration in free-tissue transfer: a review of 150 consecutive cases. Plast Reconstr Surg 1990;86(3):492–8 [discussion: 499–501].

23. Hanasono MM, Butler CE. Prevention and treatment of thrombosis in microvascular surgery. J Reconstr Microsurg 2008;24(5):305–14.

24. Esclamado RM, Carroll WR. The pathogenesis of vascular thrombosis and its impact in microvascular surgery. Head Neck 1999;21(4):355–62.

25. Rinker BD, Stewart DH, Pu LL, et al. Role of recombinant tissue plasminogen activator in free flap salvage. J Reconstr Microsurg 2007;23(2):69–73.

26. Trussler AP, Watson JP, Crisera CA. Late free-flap salvage with catheter-directed thrombolysis. Microsurgery 2008;28(4):217–22.

27. Dec W. A meta-analysis of success rates for digit replantation. Tech Hand Up Extrem Surg 2006; 10(3):124–9.

28. Waikakul S, Sakkarnkosol S, Vanadurongwan V, et al. Results of 1018 digital replantations in 552 patients. Injury 2000;31(1):33–40.

29. Brooks D, Buntic RF, Kind GM, et al. Ring avulsion: injury pattern, treatment, and outcome. Clin Plast Surg 2007;34(2):187–195, viii.

30. Lee CH, Han SK, Dhong ES, et al. The fate of microanastomosed digital arteries after successful replantation. Plast Reconstr Surg 2005;116(3): 805–10.

31. Cavadas PC. Salvage of replanted upper extremities with major soft-tissue complications. J Plast Reconstr Aesthet Surg 2007;60(7):769–75.

32. Hanel DP, Chin SH. Wrist level and proximal-upper extremity replantation. Hand Clin 2007; 23(1):13–21.

33. McCutcheon C, Hennessy B. Systemic reperfusion injury during arm replantation requiring intraoperative amputation. Anaesth Intensive Care 2002; 30(1):71–3.

34. Wood MB, Cooney WP 3rd. Above elbow limb replantation: functional results. J Hand Surg Am 1986;11(5):682–7.

35. Molski M. Replantation of fingers and hands after avulsion and crush injuries. J Plast Reconstr Aesthet Surg 2007;60(7):748–54.

36. Lykoudis EG, Papanikolaou GE, Katsikeris NF. Microvascular anastomotic aneurysms in the clinical setting: case report and review of the literature. Microsurgery 2009;29(4):293–8.

37. de Chalain TM. Exploring the use of the medicinal leech: a clinical risk-benefit analysis. J Reconstr Microsurg 1996;12(3):165–72.

38. Hayden RE, Phillips JG, McLear PW. Leeches. Objective monitoring of altered perfusion in congested flaps. Arch Otolaryngol Head Neck Surg 1988;114(12):1395–9.

39. Lee C, Mehran RJ, Lessard ML, et al. Leeches: controlled trial in venous compromised rat epigastric flaps. Br J Plast Surg 1992;45(3): 235–8.

40. Kubo T, Yano K, Hosokawa K. Management of flaps with compromised venous outflow in head and neck microsurgical reconstruction. Microsurgery 2002; 22(8):391–5.

41. Rados C. Beyond bloodletting: FDA gives leeches a medical makeover. FDA Consum 2004;38(5):9.

42. Davila VJ, Hoppe IC, Landi R, et al. The effect of anchoring sutures on medicinal leech mortality. Eplasty 2009;9:e29.

43. Granzow JW, Armstrong MB, Panthaki ZJ. A simple method for the control of medicinal leeches. J Reconstr Microsurg 2004;20(6):461–2.

44. Chepeha DB, Nussenbaum B, Bradford CR, et al. Leech therapy for patients with surgically unsalvageable venous obstruction after revascularized free tissue transfer. Arch Otolaryngol Head Neck Surg 2002;128(8):960–5.

45. Evans J, Lunnis PJ, Gaunt PN, et al. A case of septicaemia due to *Aeromonas hydrophila*. Br J Plast Surg 1990;43(3):371–2.

46. Lineaweaver WC, Hill MK, Buncke GM, et al. *Aeromonas hydrophila* infections following use of medicinal leeches in replantation and flap surgery. Ann Plast Surg 1992;29(3):238–44.

47. Whitaker IS, Kamya C, Azzopardi EA, et al. Preventing infective complications following leech therapy: is practice keeping pace with current research? Microsurgery 2009;29(8):619–25.

48. Whitaker IS, Izadi D, Oliver DW, et al. Hirudo Medicinalis and the plastic surgeon. Br J Plast Surg 2004; 57(4):348–53.

49. Nahabedian MY, Momen B, Manson PN. Factors associated with anastomotic failure after microvascular reconstruction of the breast. Plast Reconstr Surg 2004;114(1):74–82.

50. Chang DW, Reece GP, Wang B, et al. Effect of smoking on complications in patients undergoing free TRAM flap breast reconstruction. Plast Reconstr Surg 2000;105(7):2374–80.

51. Padubidri AN, Yetman R, Browne E, et al. Complications of postmastectomy breast reconstructions in smokers, ex-smokers, and nonsmokers. Plast Reconstr Surg 2001;107(2):342–9 [discussion: 350–1].

52. Howard MA, Cordeiro PG, Disa J, et al. Free tissue transfer in the elderly: incidence of perioperative complications following microsurgical reconstruction of 197 septuagenarians and octogenarians. Plast Reconstr Surg 2005;116(6):1659–68 [discussion: 1669–71].

53. Shestak KC, Jones NF. Microsurgical free-tissue transfer in the elderly patient. Plast Reconstr Surg 1991;88(2):259–63.

54. Gosain A, Chang N, Mathes S, et al. A study of the relationship between blood flow and bacterial inoculation in musculocutaneous and fasciocutaneous flaps. Plast Reconstr Surg 1990;86(6):1152–62 [discussion: 1163].

55. Mathes SJ, Alpert BS, Chang N. Use of the muscle flap in chronic osteomyelitis: experimental and clinical correlation. Plast Reconstr Surg 1982;69(5):815–29.

56. Anthony JP, Mathes SJ, Alpert BS. The muscle flap in the treatment of chronic lower extremity osteomyelitis: results in patients over 5 years after treatment. Plast Reconstr Surg 1991;88(2):311–8.

57. Yazar S, Lin CH, Lin YT, et al. Outcome comparison between free muscle and free fasciocutaneous flaps for reconstruction of distal third and ankle traumatic open tibial fractures. Plast Reconstr Surg 2006; 117(7):2468–75 [discussion: 2476–7].

58. Salgado CJ, Mardini S, Jamali AA, et al. Muscle versus nonmuscle flaps in the reconstruction of chronic osteomyelitis defects. Plast Reconstr Surg 2006;118(6):1401–11.

59. Zweifel-Schlatter M, Haug M, Schaefer DJ, et al. Free fasciocutaneous flaps in the treatment of chronic osteomyelitis of the tibia: a retrospective study. J Reconstr Microsurg 2006;22(1):41–7.

60. Musharafieh R, Osmani O, Musharafieh U, et al. Efficacy of microsurgical free-tissue transfer in chronic osteomyelitis of the leg and foot: review of 22 cases. J Reconstr Microsurg 1999;15(4):239–44.

61. Machens HG, Mailander P, Pasel J, et al. Flap perfusion after free musculocutaneous tissue transfer: the impact of postoperative complications. Plast Reconstr Surg 2000;105(7):2395–9.

62. Slavin SA, Upton J, Kaplan WD, et al. An investigation of lymphatic function following free-tissue transfer. Plast Reconstr Surg 1997;99(3):730–41 [discussion: 742–3].

Index

Note: Page numbers of article titles are in **boldface** type.

A

Aneurysm, as complication of microsurgery, 296

Antibiotics, prophylactic, in elective hand surgery, 268–270

Arthritis, adjacent, after wrist arthrodesis, 225–226
 rheumatoid, as risk factor for infection, 267
 septic, of hand and wrist, from deep-space infection, 272–273
 traumatic, of distal radioulnar joint, associated with distal radius fracture, 261–263

Arthroplasty, cemented surface replacement, 208
 of distal interphalangeal joint, 210–211
 of wrist. See *Wrist, arthroplasty of.*
 small joint, complications of, **205–212**

B

Bone anchor(s), in avulsed ligamentum subcruentum, 254, 255
 placement into ulnar fovea, 254, 256, 257

C

Carpal tunnel surgery, complex regional pain syndrome and, 287–288

Carpal tunnel syndrome, 229–230

Casting, in stiff finger, 194, 196

Cemented surface replacement arthroplasty, 208

Compartment syndrome, diagnosis of, 231
 following fractures of distal radius, 231–232
 treatment of, 231–232

Complex regional pain syndrome, after distal radius fractures, 230–231, 287
 after hand surgery, **281–289**
 complications related to, late management of, 285–286
 diagnosis of, 281
 diagnostic evaluation in, 283–284
 history and physical examination in, 282
 incidence and significance of, 281
 inspection and observation in, 282–283
 mechanical derangements and, 288
 motor testing in, 283
 oral medications in, 286
 physical examination in, 282–284
 radiologic testing in, 284
 treatment of, 284–285
 carpal tunnel surgery and, 287–288

D

Diabetes, as risk factor for infection, 266–267

Distal radioulnar joint, anatomy of, 246–248, 249
 and treatment of distal radius fractures, 246
 destabilizing injuries to triangular fibrocartilage complex, in distal radius fractures, 259
 hand function and, 245
 injury to, extensor tendon entrapment in, 233
 problems of, 217
 traumatic arthritis of, associated with distal radius fracture, 261–263

Distal radius, fractures of, compartment syndrome following, 231–232
 complex regional pain syndrome after, 287
 displaced, surgical management of ulnar side of wrist in, 251–257
 distal radius instability and stiffness as complications of, **245–264**
 ligament dysfunction in, 233–234
 neurovascular dysfunction following, 229–231
 open reduction and internal fixation of radius in, 251, 252, 259
 skin problems following, 231
 soft tisssue complications of, **229–235**
 supraphysiologic loads on triangular fibrocartilage in, 248–251
 tendon injuries associated with, 232–233
 traumatic arthritis of distal radioulnar joint and, 261–263
 treatment of, distal radioulnar joint and, 246
 failure to note anatomy of triangular fibrocartilage in, 257, 258
 instability and stiffness of, as complications of fractures of distal radius, **245–264**

Distraction plate fixation, in fractures of wrist. See *Wrist, fractures of, distraction plate fixation of.*

Dome osteotomy, in radius malunion, following distal radius fracture, 258–259

Dorsal capsulectomy, in stiff finger, 198, 200

Drains, wound closure, in hand surgery, 270–271
 to prevent infection, 271–272

Dynamic splinting, in stiff finger, 194

E

Extensor pollicus longus, rupture of, fractures of distal radius and, 232–233

Hand Clin 26 (2010) 303–306
doi:10.1016/S0749-0712(10)00028-4
0749-0712/10/$ – see front matter © 2010 Elsevier Inc. All rights reserved.

Moving?

Make sure your subscription moves with you!

To notify us of your new address, find your **Clinics Account Number** (located on your mailing label above your name), and contact customer service at:

Email: journalscustomerservice-usa@elsevier.com

800-654-2452 (subscribers in the U.S. & Canada)
314-447-8871 (subscribers outside of the U.S. & Canada)

Fax number: 314-447-8029

Elsevier Health Sciences Division
Subscription Customer Service
3251 Riverport Lane
Maryland Heights, MO 63043

*To ensure uninterrupted delivery of your subscription, please notify us at least 4 weeks in advance of move.

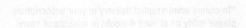